Mastering Concept-Based Teaching and Competency Assessment

3ʳᵈ EDITION

Mastering Concept-Based Teaching and Competency Assessment

A GUIDE FOR NURSE EDUCATORS

Jean Foret Giddens, PhD, RN, FAAN, ANEF

Dean and Professor
School of Nursing
Virginia Commonwealth University
Richmond, Virginia

ELSEVIER

Elsevier
3251 Riverport Lane
St. Louis, Missouri 63043

MASTERING CONCEPT-BASED TEACHING AND COMPETENCY
ASSESSMENT: A GUIDE FOR NURSE EDUCATORS,
THIRD EDITION   ISBN: 978-0-323-93445-9
Copyright © 2024 by Elsevier, Inc. All rights reserved.

Notice

Practitioners and researchers must always rely on their own experience and knowledge in evaluating and using any information, methods, compounds or experiments described herein. Because of rapid advances in the medical sciences, in particular, independent verification of diagnoses and drug dosages should be made. To the fullest extent of the law, no responsibility is assumed by Elsevier, authors, editors or contributors for any injury and/or damage to persons or property as a matter of products liability, negligence or otherwise, or from any use or operation of any methods, products, instructions, or ideas contained in the material herein.

Previous editions copyrighted 2020 and 2015.

Executive Content Strategist: Lee Henderson
Director, Content Development: Laurie K. Gower
Publishing Services Manager: Deepthi Unni
Project Manager: Sheik Mohideen K
Senior Book Designer: Margaret M. Reid

Printed in India

Last digit is the print number: 9 8 7 6 5 4 3 2 1

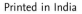

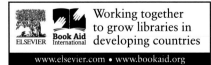

Working together
to grow libraries in
developing countries

www.elsevier.com • www.bookaid.org

Dr. Giddens earned a Bachelor of Science in Nursing from the University of Kansas, a Master of Science of Nursing from the University of Texas at El Paso, and a PhD in Education and Human Resource Studies from Colorado State University. Dr. Giddens has more than 35 years' experience in associate-degree, baccalaureate-degree, and graduate-degree nursing programs in New Mexico, Texas, Colorado, and Virginia. She is an expert in concept-based curriculum and evaluation, as well as innovative strategies for teaching and learning. Dr. Giddens has served on national nursing education taskforces, including as co-chair of the AACN Essentials Revision taskforce. She also has served as an education consultant to nursing programs throughout the United States, and is the author of multiple journal articles, electronic media, and nursing textbooks, including *Concepts for Nursing Practice.*

The education reform movement over the past two decades has been propelled by an expansion in what we know about human learning. Advances in brain research related to the process of thinking and learning have had a significant influence on the practice of teaching. Research has shown that learning is influenced by the ability to make connections between information and that such connections form knowledge structures that facilitate the application of information to multiple situations. This process is at the heart of the *conceptual approach*. Thus, the science of learning has led to the rise of the conceptual approach in primary and secondary education, as well as higher education. In recent years, significant interest in the conceptual approach has grown in nursing education. This increased interest parallels the education discipline and is seen as a way to manage excessive curriculum content through information management, to engage students, to develop the thinking skills of nursing students, and to produce highly skilled nursing graduates who can manage patients in an increasingly complex health care system.

The conceptual approach represents the incorporation of concepts, exemplars, concept-based curriculum, concept-based instruction, conceptual learning, and competency assessment into the practice of nurse educators. For most faculty, the conceptual approach represents a considerable change in the way the curriculum is structured and taught. It requires a collective reframing of the education process among faculty and students. Although there is significant interest in adopting the conceptual approach in nursing programs, many faculty groups have not had adequate exposure to this approach or clear guidance and therefore lack the expertise or understanding. They may have teaching expertise but just not in conceptual teaching, which is needed for optimal success.

This book was written specifically as a resource for the conceptual approach in nursing education. Targeted users of this book include nursing faculty in undergraduate or graduate nursing programs and graduate nursing students who are preparing for a career in academia. This book does not attempt to replicate the many excellent resources that exist related to general education on faculty roles, teaching strategies, and curriculum development. However, this book does present these topics within the context of the conceptual approach. It is also not expected that an individual will read this book sequentially from cover to cover—so each chapter stands alone and is beneficial in relation to the desired topic area.

1. Chapter 1 focuses on the conceptual approach as a general overview. It is an excellent starting point for faculty who want a broad "30,000-foot" view of the conceptual approach and the various elements.
2. Chapter 2 presents a discussion of competencies in nursing education. Specifically, a discussion regarding how the competency-based approach differs from the conceptual approach is presented and, perhaps more importantly, confirms the application of competency assessment as a component of the conceptual approach.
3. Chapter 3 provides a deep look into concepts and understanding what is meant by concept analysis. This chapter is presented from a theoretical lens and is intended to

deepen the understanding of concepts; this understanding is foundational to the conceptual approach.

4. Chapter 4 provides a discussion about how to develop a concept-based curriculum. Although this process mirrors any other curriculum development process, concepts are used as the infrastructure for the curriculum, and this chapter explains how.

5. Chapter 5 offers readers a look into what is now known about how the human brain learns and how the use of concepts enhances learning.

6. Chapter 6 presents a discussion of conceptual teaching for the classroom setting and how this differs from traditional content-focused instruction. Furthermore, the reader is provided examples of specific teaching strategies that result in conceptual learning.

7. Chapter 7 presents a discussion of conceptual teaching in the clinical setting and how examples-focused learning activities focused on concepts.

8. Chapter 8 presents an overview of evaluation strategies that faculty can use to determine achievement of student learning—again with a specific emphasis on conceptual learning and competency assessment.

9. Chapter 9 provides the reader with an overview of the nursing literature as it relates to the conceptual approach and suggestions for developing expertise in the conceptual approach.

It is important to note that the nine chapters in this book are closely interrelated to one another. In other words, some overlap is unavoidable. For example, part of the development and implementation of a concept-based curriculum (Chapter 4) includes the development of teaching strategies (Chapters 6 and 7) and the evaluation of learning (Chapter 8). As another example, the development of effective teaching strategies (Chapters 6 and 7) requires the foundational understanding of concepts (Chapter 3) and an understanding of human learning with concepts (Chapter 5).

It is my hope that this book serves as a useful resource for faculty who are courageous enough to embark on the conceptual approach journey and for graduate nursing students preparing for a career in academic nursing. I hope this book will serve you well along the way!

Jean Foret Giddens

ACKNOWLEDGMENTS

It has been my honor and privilege to advance the conceptual approach in nursing. This work has been enhanced through collaborations with a number of colleagues across the country. I am particularly grateful to my two colleagues, Dr. Linda Caputi and Dr. Beth Rodgers, who were involved with the two previous editions of this book. Their extraordinary expertise has led to deepening of my own conceptual understandings. I also extend my gratitude and appreciation to my colleagues at Elsevier, Lee Henderson, a long-time colleague and advocate, and Laurie Gower, who helped me stay on schedule and navigated our work through production.

I would be remiss not to mention the incredible patience and love from my husband, Jay Corazza. His support and tolerance of my obsession to write and create, and my involvement in other professional opportunities are remarkable and deeply appreciated.

Lastly, I extend my sincere gratitude to my nursing faculty colleagues for moving our profession forward. May the torch burn long and bright!

Jean Foret Giddens

CONTENTS

CHAPTER 1

The Conceptual Approach— Background and Benefits

If you have been a nurse educator anytime during the past 15 years, you have likely noticed significant movement toward the conceptual approach as a basis for curriculum design and teaching. Perhaps you heard about this approach at a conference or from a colleague or read about it in a journal article. One or more faculty members from your nursing program may have discussed the possibility of adopting a concept-based curriculum as part of a curriculum redesign. Perhaps some faculty in your program are exploring the conceptual approach to support competency-based assessment. Perhaps you are part of a faculty group that is actively developing or implementing a concept-based curriculum. You may also be a new faculty member in a program that offers a concept-based curriculum. Regardless of how or where you have heard about it, the conceptual approach has been an important trend in nursing education that has grown exponentially.

You may be wondering if the conceptual approach really represents nursing education transformation or merely a trend that will pass. Indeed, educators should be careful not to jump on every bandwagon that comes along. In many cases, education innovations gain immediate interest but are quickly abandoned when implementation proves challenging and/or when outcomes fall short of expectations. Nurse educators have very full workloads and must make the best use of their time. Thus, regarding any trend, educators are encouraged to consider what is reasonable and supported by education science.

A conceptual approach in nursing education may be adopted for many reasons. Among the most important reasons are the management of excessive curriculum content, engagement of students in the learning process, helping students develop advanced thinking skills leading to clinical judgment, and graduating highly competent nursing students who are skilled in the management of patients. Successful adoption and implementation of the conceptual approach requires nurse educators to transform the learning environment from the traditional teacher-focused delivery of information to a student-centered environment in which students are actively engaged in the learning process. Carrieri-Kohlman et al. (2003) describe the conceptual approach as "a process that deliberately attempts to examine the nature and substance of nursing from a conceptual perspective" (p. 1). For most nursing programs, the conceptual approach represents a cultural shift in the way faculty and students perceive their roles in the teaching-learning process. The purpose of this chapter is to provide historic background regarding concept-based approaches in education and nursing, describe what is meant by the *conceptual approach*, and present benefits of the conceptual approach for contemporary nursing education.

Background

Many nurse educators might be surprised to learn that the conceptual approach is not a new trend but rather has been borrowed from other disciplines and adapted to nursing. Two interesting historical perspectives are associated with the conceptual approach—one from the education discipline and the other from nursing.

THE EARLY YEARS

In the education discipline, curriculum design was historically approached through discrete areas and topical organizers. The emphasis of curriculum development was on the selection and organization of content around the topical organizers (such as math, social studies, sciences, etc.) with educational objectives primarily targeting basic knowledge acquisition. Student learning focused on memorization of facts and the practice of discrete skills. As an example, a traditional approach to learning the mathematic skill of multiplication involves memorizing columns of multiplication equations with answers. Other examples include memorizing rules of grammar or memorizing all 50 state capitals. This is not to say that rote learning does not have benefits; the ability to recall basic facts provides a necessary foundation for conceptual learning. However, rote learning and memorization do not develop active thinking necessary for higher-level problem solving.

As early as the 1950s, Hilda Taba, a visionary educator from San Francisco, proposed the idea of concepts (as opposed to topics) as content organizers. She emphasized developing the capability of discriminating essential from nonessential information. In her work, concepts are referred to as high-level abstractions, and she proposed inductive strategies for concept formation. Taba postulated that a person's understanding of a concept expands when challenged with increasingly complex examples representing the concept (Taba, 1966). At that time, critics of her work raised concerns about the abstract nature of concepts. It was recognized that unless concepts were clearly defined, they were challenging for faculty to teach in a clear and efficient way.

During this same general time period, many grand theories were emerging in the nursing discipline, such as those proposed by Abdellah, Johnson, Rogers, Orem, King, and Roy (Alligood, 2022). The era of grand theories reflected the maturing of nursing as a distinct discipline. Nursing grand theories represent the organization, arrangement, or framework of key concepts and principles that describe the profession. These theories provided a mechanism for the nursing profession to clearly establish itself as a unique and separate health care discipline. Defining professional identity is important work for any profession on its continuum of ongoing development. Subsequently, in the 1970s and 1980s, the design of nursing curricula based on a grand theory became common practice. Because concepts associated with the chosen theory were often used as the foundation for the curriculum, many of these curricula were referred to as "concept based." For example, Orem's Self-Care Framework (Orem, 1971) was widely used as a basis for curriculum development. Orem's theory included the following concepts:

- Self-care
- Self-care agency
- Therapeutic self-care demand
- Self-care deficit
- Nursing agency
- Nursing system

These concepts serve as the building blocks of Orem's theory and are very useful in that context. However, use of these as foundational concepts for a nursing curriculum was problematic for many nursing programs when faculty did not clearly understand the concepts and did not know how to teach conceptually or how to link specific content to the concepts. Although nursing faculty in some schools were successful with this type of curriculum design, many educators struggled to translate abstract theoretical concepts to practical application, particularly when teaching novice learners. Interestingly, some of these same issues were experienced within the education discipline.

EDUCATION REFORM

It was not until the 1990s that significant education reform propelled the idea of different models of curricula and different approaches to teaching. In a study of science and mathematics education, authors described curricula in the United States as "an inch deep and a mile wide" (Schmidt et al. 1997). It became increasingly obvious to educators that the massive content covered in education was limiting true cognitive development (Erikson, 2002). At the same time, increased attention was being directed at research into human learning. In the late 1990s, the National Research Council conducted a study that led to the publication of *How People Learn* (Bransford et al., 2000), which provided a synthesis on the science of learning. Bransford and colleagues noted a convergence of evidence across many disciplines, with significant implications for education. Advances in brain research related to the process of thinking and learning have influenced teaching, curriculum design, instructional assessment, and learning environments. As a result, an emphasis on linking brain research (and the research of learning) to teaching practice has increased. One of the themes noted from the research is the notion that learning is influenced by students' ability to make connections between information. Structural changes in the brain occur through a process called *neuroplasticity*—in other words, neurons build connections in response to learning. These neurological connections form knowledge structures that allow learners to apply information and knowledge effectively to multiple situations—including new situations. This process is at the heart of the conceptual approach. Thus, the science of learning has influenced the rise of a concept-based curriculum as an alternative to the traditional curriculum models in primary and secondary education (Erikson, 2002; Erickson et al., 2017).

THE CONCEPTUAL APPROACH IN NURSING EDUCATION

Although nursing was slower to embrace changes in teaching and curriculum design, many nurse educators took cues from the education discipline. They became aware of the science supporting new models for teaching and learning, and they reexamined concept-based approaches. The current conceptual approach movement in nursing began in the mid-2000s. Unlike concept-based curricula of the past (which were largely based on a single grand theory), contemporary concept-based models in nursing education feature common concepts that have emerged from nursing science as the profession has matured. The expansion of concepts presented in the context of nursing is reflected in the nursing literature, particularly during the last 30 years. Thus, the primary distinctions in present-day concept-based models in nursing compared with those of the past are that (1) more concepts have been defined and formally developed, (2) the concepts are less abstract (and easier for faculty and students to understand), and (3) advances in the science of teaching and learning are applied.

MISCONCEPTIONS AND CLARIFICATIONS

Misconception: The conceptual approach is a new idea from the nursing discipline that is spreading to other disciplines.

Clarification: The conceptual approach was proposed in the 1950s with origins in primary and secondary education. Today it is applied in many disciplines and levels of education.

The Conceptual Approach

Because many ideas and terms are used to describe the conceptual approach in nursing education, clarification is important as a starting point. The term *conceptual approach* in education is broad and represents the incorporation of the following separate but interrelated elements: concepts, exemplars, concept-based curriculum, concept-based instruction, conceptual learning, and evaluation of student learning (Box 1.1). These elements are briefly described here and will be expanded on in various chapters throughout this text.

ELEMENTS OF THE CONCEPTUAL APPROACH

Concepts

Central to the conceptual approach are concepts. A concept is an organizing idea or mental construct represented by common attributes. Rodgers describes concepts as "an abstraction that is expressed in some form" (1989, p. 332). Key terms to focus on in the two concept descriptions above are *mental construct* and

---

BOX 1.1 ■ Elements of the Conceptual Approach

- **Concept:** An organizing idea or mental image composed of attributes.
- **Exemplar:** A specific topic or an example represented by the concept.
- **Concept-Based Curriculum:** A curriculum that is designed by organizing content around key concepts.
- **Concept-Based Instruction:** An instructional process featuring student-centered learning activities that focuses on concepts and the application of information to concepts.
- **Conceptual Learning:** A process by which learners develop high-level thinking skills and the ability to apply facts in the context of related concepts.
- **Evaluation of Learning**: The method by which faculty evaluate student attainment of conceptual learning outcomes and/or competencies.

---

abstraction. Important to note is that a concept is not a physical object—you can't directly see, touch, taste, or smell a concept. Concepts are ideas or the organization of thoughts formed in the mind that have been described as the natural bridge between the world" (Rosch, 1999, p. 61). Concepts are often represented by physical things. For example, the concept of *Fruit* is a mental construct we all share. Physical objects that represent the concept of fruit include apples, oranges, and bananas. Put another way, you can't eat the concept of *Fruit*, but a bowl of strawberries (which represents the concept of *Fruit*) is delicious! However, such distinctions are not always so simple. Some concepts do not have any physical objects to represent them. For example, the concept of *Beauty* is more abstract than the concept of *Fruit* because of the variability in the interpretation of beauty. *Beauty* can be associated with objects (such as flowers or jewelry) or less tangible things such as landscapes, personality, or a spiritual experience. In other words, for some concepts, the exemplars are abstractions in themselves.

In the conceptual approach, concepts form the infrastructure of a concept-based curriculum and are the key elements associated with concept-based instruction, conceptual learning, and evaluation. Concepts represent the key ideas that are used to organize knowledge, facts, skills, and competencies across multiple situations and contexts. Concepts function as hubs for transferable knowledge.

Any given discipline, including nursing, contains an endless number of concepts that range from the very broad (known as *macroconcepts*) to the narrow (known as *microconcepts*). Several concepts can link to each macroconcept, and several microconcepts can link to each concept (Fig. 1.1). The designation of macroconcept, concept, and microconcept is context specific. In other words, what is considered a concept for undergraduate nursing education might be considered a macroconcept for an expert in a given area; likewise, what is considered an advanced or microconcept for an undergraduate student may be considered a basic concept to an expert. For example, *Ethics* is widely considered an appropriate concept for nursing education. As a way to frame the scope of *Ethics* as a concept, four ethical principles—autonomy, beneficence, nonmaleficence, and

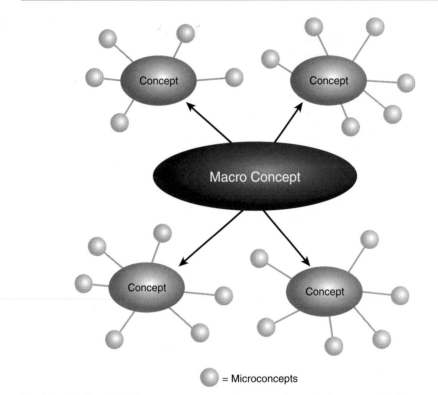

Fig. 1.1   Relationship between macroconcepts, concepts, and microconcepts. Macroconcepts are broad and abstract with multiple associated concepts. Microconcepts are narrow, specific, and tend to be associated with specialty practice/knowledge.

justice—might be used. However, an advanced scholar and expert in this area might consider *Ethics* as a macro concept, with four primary concepts: *Autonomy, Beneficence, Nonmaleficence,* and *Justice.* Thus, a crucial task of educators who adopt the conceptual approach is to not only identify and clearly address key concepts to be used, but also ensure that the appropriate level of concept is selected for the learner.

Not only should concepts be selected based on relevancy to the discipline and the program of study, but they also should be organized logically within the curriculum and be used consistently by faculty for maximum benefit to the learner. Achieving such consistency among faculty requires a solid understanding (and agreement) of how the concepts are to be used in the curriculum across courses, how to present the concepts in a useful way to students, and how to link essential content knowledge to the concepts for in-depth understanding. Additionally, faculty must help students recognize the relationships among the key concepts, because in most clinical situations several concepts are involved (which are referred to as *interrelated concepts*). For example, Fig. 1.2 shows the concept *Health Promotion* and several key interrelated concepts. In this example, three different concept categories are represented: *Health and Illness* (at the right), *Professional*

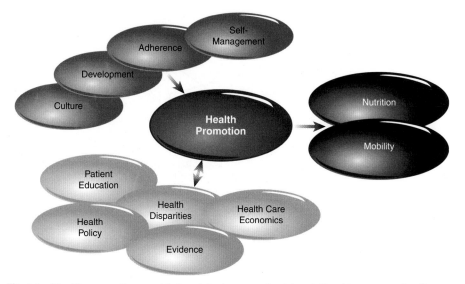

Fig. 1.2 **Health promotion and interrelated concepts.** Interrelationships among health care recipient concepts, health and illness concepts, and professional nursing concepts. (From Giddens J. *Concepts for Nursing Practice.* 3rd ed. St. Louis, MO: Elsevier; 2021.)

Nursing (at bottom, *left*), and *Health Care Recipient* (*top*). Each of these interrelated concepts not only link to health promotion but also link to each other (as illustrated by the arrows). Interrelated concept diagrams help visualize the interrelationships and illustrate the complexity of concepts. Concepts are discussed in greater detail in Chapter 3.

Exemplars

Exemplars represent specific examples of a topic. For a concept-based curriculum, the exemplars are the most important examples, topics, or content related to a concept. Typically there are many exemplars for any given concept, and exemplars usually connect to multiple concepts. In other words, a concept is not represented by only one exemplar, and an exemplar can represent many very different concepts. For example, returning to the previous example of *Fruit* as a concept, many types of *Fruit* could be used as exemplars including apples and strawberries. However, apples and strawberries could also be used as exemplars of the concept of red.

In nursing, exemplars are an essential component of the conceptual approach because they represent essential content knowledge. It is worth noting that facts and base knowledge remain important components of learning. Facts represent specific information embedded within exemplars; thus students build conceptual understandings based on an accurate knowledgebase. The complex interrelationship between facts/topics, exemplars, concepts, and macroconcepts is at the heart of gaining conceptual understandings. Fig. 1.3 illustrates this complex relationship. Exemplars provide specific context and help students grasp a deep

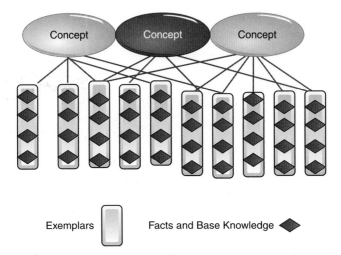

Fig. 1.3 Concepts, exemplars, and facts. The relationship between facts, exemplars, and concepts is complex.

understanding of the concept. In nursing, exemplars can be health-related conditions experienced by patients (such as asthma, a hip fracture, or an allergic reaction); situations experienced by patients and families in the context of health (such as death and dying, caregiver roles, developmental delays, and bullying); or situations experienced by nurses in the context of professional nursing practice (such as informed consent, delegation of care, medication teaching, and quality improvement projects).

One of the fundamental tasks of nurse educators who are adopting the conceptual approach is to identify the exemplars to be used for each concept. Faculty members often feel compelled to include multiple exemplars for each concept (often content from their own specialty or content they have traditionally taught) because of their belief that the content is critical and that students must know it. However, one of the benefits of the conceptual approach is information management, and thus the exemplars should be limited to those most representative or important in helping students attain a grasp of the concept. The learning emphasis should be on the development of cognitive connections back to the concept— in other words, the student should not only learn about the exemplar, but how it relates back to one or more concepts. Because exemplars typically link to multiple concepts, faculty should incorporate exemplars in the curriculum plan in such a way that repetitious use of a particular exemplar is avoided. For example, pneumonia could be used effectively as an exemplar for the concepts of gas exchange, infection, acid-base balance, or fatigue. However, it would be unwise to use pneumonia four times within the curriculum as an exemplar, especially considering the many other key content areas that students need to learn. Faculty must help students make purposeful cognitive connections from the exemplar to the primary concept and to other key interrelated concepts. This is a necessary step to avoid information overload.

Concept-Based Curriculum

A third element of the conceptual approach is a concept-based curriculum, in which concepts serve as "foundational organizers" that provide an infrastructure to the curriculum. A concept-based curriculum represents a major paradigm shift for nursing because it moves away from an emphasis on content and toward an emphasis on concepts and conceptual learning (Giddens and Brady, 2007). Featured concepts within the courses serve as cornerstones for concept-based instruction and conceptual learning (Giddens et al., 2008). Lynn Erikson, a leading expert in concept-based curriculum and instruction, describes the differences between content-focused and concept-focused curricula as "the difference between memorizing facts related to the American Revolution and developing and sharing ideas related to the concepts of freedom and independence as a result of studying the American Revolution" (Erikson, 2002, p. 50).

When a concept-based curriculum is designed, several key decisions must be made. As with any curriculum, faculty should first determine desired program learning outcomes and competencies. After this initial step, concept categories or an organizing framework should be developed, and concepts should be selected. Each concept should be developed so that faculty members gain a shared understanding about what the concept means and what it represents. Exemplars that will be linked to each concept also must be chosen. Exemplar selection should be based on the best examples of the concept or the most common situations represented. Next, decisions regarding the type of courses and the arrangement of concepts within courses must be made, followed by the actual development of each course, and the plan for teaching within the course. Curriculum development also includes a general plan for evaluation to ensure that students attain program learning outcomes and competence. Implementation issues include faculty development, student orientation, and maintaining the curriculum integrity. These key decisions and issues are summarized in Box 1.2 and are described further in Chapter 4.

Concept-Based Instruction

A fourth element associated with the conceptual approach is concept-based instruction. This instructional process is characterized by student-centered learning activities that focus on *target concepts* (meaning the featured concept for a unit

---

BOX 1.2 ■ Key Steps and Decisions When Designing a Concept-Based Curriculum

- Review mission, vision, and values of institution/school.
- Develop program outcomes and competencies.
- Develop an organizing framework for concepts.
- Select and develop featured curriculum concepts.
- Identify exemplars for each concept.
- Organize concepts and exemplars into courses/course development.
- Develop a program evaluation plan.

of study) and the application of key exemplars to concepts. It is worth mentioning again that the focus of instruction is on both the concept (such as a concept overview) *and* the specific exemplars linked to that concept.

How does one actually teach a concept? A typical starting point is the concept overview (or concept presentation). A concept overview includes the concept definition, scope or categories of the concept, concept attributes, assessment, process and consequences, and nursing management. Faculty incorporate important facts and information as foundational knowledge to the concept. As an example, students must understand learning domains (cognitive domain, psychomotor domain, and affective domain), as well as educational approaches, before they can grasp the concept of patient education. The use of facts in foundational information is absolutely necessary as part of the conceptual learning process because base knowledge supports conceptual learning; conceptual learning leads to conceptual understanding, which facilitates the students' ability to make generalizations.

The concept overview is followed by the application of exemplars to deepen the students' understanding of the concept. A deep understanding of the concept leads to the ability of the student to form generalizations and relationships between concepts. It is also important to note that there is not a single or specific instructional strategy for conceptual teaching. Concept-based instruction incorporates a variety of teaching strategies and learning experiences that require higher levels of thinking from faculty and students (Erikson, 2008). Ideally, students are placed in learning groups and work through cases, situations, questions, or problems posed by the instructor as opposed to faculty-centered lectures on concepts. Chapters 6 and 7 are devoted to concept-based instructional strategies that support conceptual learning.

Conceptual Learning

Conceptual learning is an active process that engages students and results in synergistic thinking. Timpson and Bendel-Simso (1996) described conceptual learning as a process through which students learn to organize information into logical mental structures and become increasingly skilled at thinking. During the learning process, students link factual information and exemplars to concepts. Students gain an understanding of the concept through a concept overview and then by actively applying information learned to the concept—and making cognitive links and generalizations to other information. The desired learning outcome is an in-depth understanding of the concept and the ability to transfer ideas to other situations through these cognitive connections. Faculty should be aware, however, that learners must have accurate baseline understandings of information on which to build. Students with inaccurate understanding of information will build on these, leading to further inaccuracies as learning occurs. For this reason, there is value in reviewing and clarifying previously learned information. In nursing, learning experiences ideally should be placed in the context of a clinical situation and should be purposeful; in other words, learners should clearly recognize the benefit of what they are learning as it pertains to the practice of nursing. Engagement in learning is enhanced when students perceive learning as purposeful and they can see a direct application to their area of study (Ambrose et al., 2010; Bransford et al., 2000; Sousa, 2010). Conceptual learning is presented in greater depth in Chapter 5.

Evaluation of Learning

The final element of the conceptual approach is the evaluation of student learning. Learning assessment is not unique to the conceptual approach, as this is a component of all educational approaches. That said, assessment of conceptual learning requires intentional metrics or indicators to determine if the student learned the information associated with the concept, and if the learner can apply that learning into a situational context. In nursing, this means translating what has been learned into clinical practice. Evaluation should include confirmation of knowledge acquisition, comprehension, and application and is accomplished through a combination of traditional assessment strategies. An increasingly common way to evaluate learning in the health sciences is through competency assessment (Lucey, 2018), particularly in the clinical learning environment. Competencies are observable and measurable outcome statements that describe what a learner can do with what they know. As educators adopt the conceptual approach, the incorporation of competencies into the conceptual framework for learner assessment is an important component to consider.

MISCONCEPTIONS AND CLARIFICATIONS	
Misconception: The conceptual approach occurs as a result of designing and implementing a concept-based curriculum.	**Clarification:** The conceptual approach is attained with the adoption of a concept-based curriculum (using concepts and exemplars) and the practice of concept-based instruction to optimize conceptual learning.

COHESIVENESS OF THE ELEMENTS

The Greek philosopher Aristotle is credited with coining the phrase, "The whole is greater than the sum of its parts." This phrase captures the significance of the conceptual approach as a cohesive, comprehensive plan as opposed to a loose collection of one or more elements. The conceptual approach requires an intentional and planned process whereby concepts influence curriculum design, teaching, learning, and evaluation. This distinction is important because the incorporation of all six elements (see Box 1.1) is necessary for a successful concept-based educational platform. Although each element stands on its own, a powerful synergistic effect occurs when all the elements are meaningfully incorporated into an education plan. Successful adoption of the conceptual approach in nursing requires a commitment among faculty to follow a concept-based curriculum and to learn how to teach conceptually through carefully designed instructional strategies. Students should be actively engaged in the learning process by applying content in purposeful ways and by learning to make cognitive connections to concepts. The end goal is for learners to gain a deep understanding of the concept and acquire the ability to transfer ideas to other concepts and contexts. This outcome represents the higher-level thinking skills necessary for sound clinical judgment in patient care settings. Consider the following two scenarios:

Scenario 1

Faculty members of an undergraduate nursing program work very hard to develop a concept-based curriculum. As part of this process, they write learning outcomes and core competencies, identify key nursing concepts from the literature, agree on exemplars, and develop courses around the concepts. Although some of the faculty members attempt to incorporate more student-centered learning activities in their approach to teaching, the majority continue to use the traditional lecture format and focus primarily on exemplars with little to no linkage to the concepts. Additionally, several faculty members become concerned about the loss of what they consider to be "essential information" and add content back into their courses.

Scenario 2

Janice teaches a nursing skills course in a nursing program that has not undergone a significant curriculum revision in 15 years. After attending a conference presentation on conceptual teaching and learning, Janice decides to adopt a concept-based instructional approach for her course. She identifies key concepts for each unit and uses student-centered teaching strategies to help students link their course content and skills to concepts within her course. Students enrolled in Janice's course find that her teaching strategies are different from those of other faculty. Although most students like the way the course is taught, some students complain because Janice does not give them the information they need for the course examinations.

In the first scenario, faculty undoubtedly spent significant time and energy to redesign the curriculum and are proud to have a concept-based curriculum. However, two primary elements associated with the conceptual approach are missing: a lack of commitment among faculty to adopt concept-based instruction, and a lost opportunity for students to benefit from a conceptual learning experience. The fact that some faculty members elected to add additional content into their courses further undermines the benefit of adopting a concept-based curriculum.

In the second scenario, Janice is motivated to change her teaching methods. By incorporating student-centered learning activities into her teaching plan, Janice is becoming increasingly comfortable with and skilled in concept-based instruction. She is also providing an engaging learning environment that is enjoyed by most students in her course. However, because no mechanism is in place for students to encounter the concepts in other courses within the curriculum, the experience occurs in isolation with limited effect.

Although the specific situation in each scenario is different, both scenarios are similar in that one or more elements of the conceptual approach were adopted. However, long-term benefits are unlikely to be achieved because one or more key elements of the conceptual approach were not incorporated. Does this mean that complete consensus must be achieved among faculty before they adopt the conceptual approach for their nursing programs? Absolutely not! Gaining complete consensus among any faculty group is unrealistic because of the very nature of academe. A diversity of perspectives, opinions, and values is expected in all organizations. However, for successful adoption of the conceptual approach, critical mass is needed; in other words, adequate support must exist among faculty who teach in the program and from the school's administrative leadership.

Benefits of the Conceptual Approach

We are in the midst of widespread change regarding what is known about human learning. What started as a trickle effect has become a force that is changing the landscape of education. The education of students in all disciplines—including nursing—is being dramatically influenced by these events. The conceptual approach links well with this change and offers multiple known benefits, which include addressing content saturation and information management and preparing nurses to successfully practice in complex health care environments by developing conceptual thinking skills that lead to good clinical judgment and collaboration.

ADDRESSING CONTENT SATURATION

Most educators agree that one of their greatest challenges is having sufficient time to teach all the curriculum content. Concerns about excessive curriculum content have appeared in the nursing literature for over two decades (Deane and Asselin, 2015; Diekelmann, 2002; Diekelmann and Smythe, 2004; Forbes and Hickey, 2009; Giddens and Brady, 2007; Hendricks and Wangerin, 2017; Ironside, 2004; National League for Nursing, 2003; Royal and Zakrajsek, 2017). Excessive content can be partly attributable to what has been known as the "information age." The exponential generation of new information makes it impossible not only to teach everything that is known in a given discipline but also to keep up with advances and changes in what was previously known. It has been estimated that as much as 50% of the information learned in a 4-year degree program changes within 2 years after graduation. This issue is exacerbated by the traditional "instructor-centric" approach to teaching. Faculty who subscribe to this perspective believe they must "cover" all the content, and the common belief is that students cannot be expected to know anything unless it has been specifically taught in a course. This expectation is quite a burden for any faculty member to carry! With this perspective, classroom time typically becomes little more than information delivery sessions as opposed to learning sessions. Excessive curriculum content has also coincided with the increased size of nursing textbooks (because of the increased generation of nursing knowledge). Many faculty feel obligated to cover large amounts of the information found in textbooks rather than encouraging students to use these books as a learning resource and reference. It is easy to see how the cycle perpetuates the problem. The conceptual approach alleviates the issue of content saturation by limiting the number of concepts and exemplars used and by emphasizing students' ability to make linkages to content to which they are exposed, even if it has not been through formal learning activities within the curriculum. The adage "less is more" applies here, not only in terms of the delivery of content, but more importantly, in the result of better learning.

INFORMATION MANAGEMENT

A curriculum focused on content generally emphasizes student memorization of facts (as they are known at that point in time) and does little to prepare students to manage the large volume of changing information they will encounter not only as students but also throughout their career. Information management refers to the ability to *locate, analyze, interpret*, and *apply* new information to specific situations. Because it is impossible for any health care professional to know all the information needed to care for all patients, health care professionals must be highly skilled in information management as a basis for evidence-based care. Nursing education must shift from information delivery to the creation of learning environments in which students are required to locate, analyze, interpret, and apply information as part of learning within classroom, laboratory, and clinical environments. These elements are also foundational to conceptual learning. The conceptual approach fosters students' development of information management by learning to link new and emerging information to concept structures and apply the information to a variety of contexts. These elements are described in the following sections, and an example is provided in Box 1.3.

Locate Information

Health care professionals must know how and where to efficiently locate accurate information on which to base their practice. More specifically, this ability means knowing appropriate and reliable sources (e.g., practice, policy, or procedure guidelines and evidence-based practice findings) and having the skill to access these sources (such as through the Internet, Intranet, or a resource manual).

BOX 1.3 ■ Exemplar: Information Management in Practice

Terrin, a nurse working in an inpatient unit, has an order to administer a new pharmacologic agent with which he is unfamiliar. He is told that the agent has only been available for use for 6 months. Terrin logs onto the hospital Intranet website (*locate*) to review the drug information and administration guidelines. Terrin carefully reads the drug information and notices that there are two indications for using the agent; he also notes that the administration guidelines are dependent on many variables, including intended use, age, weight, and underlying medical conditions (*analyze*). Based on the information presented, Terrin gains an understanding regarding the specific context for which the agent was ordered (*interpret*). He uses this information to administer the agent correctly and to monitor the patient for potential adverse effects (*apply*).

Analyze Information

Analysis of information requires a critical examination of information elements to determine the relationship of the parts or to discover meaning. New information and the supporting evidence are often complex, requiring careful consideration of all elements. Health care professionals must be able to gain an accurate understanding of new information through analysis of the information that is available. With the extensive amount of information (and misinformation) available on the Internet, nurses must be capable of critiquing information to determine accuracy and relevance.

Interpret Information

The process of information analysis should lead to the ability of the health care professional to draw meaning from the information. One aspect of the process is to analyze the information, but a key component is the ability to translate the information into understandable terms or context. The process of interpretation means gaining an understanding of the meaning or significance of the information. This process means gaining an understanding of how the information fits with the context of care within the clinical environment.

Apply Information

The evidence-based practice movement ultimately is about applying the latest evidence or information to one's practice. Application of information refers to the process of putting newly learned or discovered information to use. It is assumed that the newly discovered/learned information comes from a reliable source. In the context of health care, the information must be applied correctly to provide evidence-based care.

STUDENT LEARNING AND ENGAGEMENT

Another significant benefit of the conceptual approach is the emphasis on student learning as opposed to the instruction provided by faculty. By and large, the emphasis in education has been on what the instructor does; this notion is captured very well by Bellack, who noted that "...nursing education continues to be 'teaching heavy' and 'learning light'" (Bellack, 2008, p. 439). With the conceptual approach, learning occurs when students develop skills in building cognitive connections to previous learning as opposed to learning facts. As a result, learners become more effective and efficient thinkers and problem solvers.

Effective, coordinated health care delivery depends on collaboration among health care professionals. Teamwork and Collaboration, one of the six core competencies from Quality and Safety Education for Nurses (QSEN), emphasizes the need for nurses to be skilled collaborators, not only with other nurses but also with persons from other disciplines (Quality and Safety Education for Nurses, n.d.). Teams and Teamwork is also a core competency identified by the Interprofessional Education Collaborative Expert Panel (IPEC, 2011). Thus, there is little doubt that graduates of nursing programs need a strong foundation in collaboration. Collaborative learning is at the heart of the conceptual approach. Historically, higher education has rewarded individual achievement, and this perspective is reinforced in a traditional classroom, where students take in information and are tested on the content. The conceptual approach requires students to learn in groups, and thus collaborative learning in school translates well to collaboration in clinical practice. If nurse educators are sincere in setting expectations that nursing graduates "play well with others," then collaborative learning must occur as a part of the education process from the first to last semesters.

In addition to facilitating collaborative learning, the conceptual approach also provides a platform to design interprofessional learning activities, events, and courses. Most concepts found in a nursing curriculum actually apply to all health care disciplines. For example, students enrolled in medicine, nursing, pharmacy, dentistry, or physical therapy all must learn about concepts such as *Culture, Ethics, Health Promotion, Informatics, Quality, Safety, Infection,* and *Gas Exchange.* Even though many of these concepts have universal application, each discipline plays a unique role in the provision of health care as it relates to the concepts. The conceptual approach provides a unique opportunity for the development of a robust core interprofessional curriculum featuring collaborative learning and team-based care across disciplines.

FROM CONCEPTUAL THINKING TO CLINICAL JUDGMENT

Nursing graduates must develop skill in clinical reasoning and clinical judgment for success in an increasingly complex health care environment. The linear approach to learning in traditional content-focused curricula does little to facilitate skills needed by nurses in the complex health care system. Tanner's model of clinical judgment (Tanner, 2006) illustrates that a nurse's response to a clinical situation is influenced by his or her previous experiences with regard to a situation, noticing when patterns are inconsistent with a given situation (i.e., taking into consideration the context of the situation), and correctly interpreting and clarifying information (Fig. 1.4). Several studies have shown an association between concept-based learning and the development of clinical judgment and clinical reasoning (Alfayoumi, 2019, Gonzalez, 2018; Lasater and Nielsen, 2009; Nielsen, 2009, 2016). Conceptual thinking skills facilitates clinical judgment and clinical reasoning because of the cognitive connections to concepts made by students when encountering new information. Having an in-depth understanding of a concept provides the necessary platform for students and practicing nurses.

BUILDING DISCIPLINARY UNDERSTANDING

A focus on concepts and conceptual learning makes it possible to take the knowledge that the nurse possesses and look at it in the abstract, outside of an immediate application, initially, thus helping to recognize that there is thought and cognitive power in the concept. That thought or knowledge then can be applied to nursing situations that include patient care or other health-related foci.

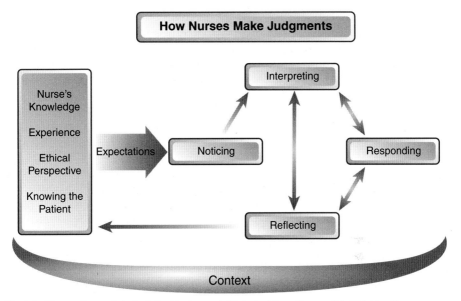

Fig. 1.4   Tanner's model of clinical judgment. (Adapted from Tanner CA. Thinking like a nurse: a research-based model of clinical judgment in nursing. *J Nurs Educ*. 2006;45(60):204–211.)

A nurse with a strong conceptual grasp of the discipline understands their role beyond describing tasks. He or she would talk about the creation of empathic relationships with care recipients, whether they be individuals, families, or communities. A nurse who works with persons who have chronic heart disease, for example, would not answer a question about nursing by saying, "I explain their medications, teach them about pacing their activities, and tell them how to monitor their weight." Instead, the nurse can describe work with this population by discussing concepts such as *Mobility*, *Gas Exchange*, and *Self-Management* to help the patient adjust his or her activities to achieve a level of independence and quality of life that is consistent with individual life goals and physiological capacities. The nurse also could relay that he or she has a strong grasp of the illness trajectory and the threats to identity that often accompany chronic illness and, rather than focusing primarily on monitoring for medication adherence and physiological stability or deterioration, works with an understanding of what it is like to live with a chronic condition to help the patient maintain dignity and self-worth. The nurse also would understand the importance of social support in such a situation and work with the patient to develop appropriate strategies to achieve reasonable goals in the situation. Such a description would be quite a change from how a nurse otherwise might describe this type of work, perhaps saying merely, "I work with people who have heart disease."

This approach sometimes is confused with "holism," an important aspect of nursing and one of the characteristics that differentiates it from other disciplines. A holistic focus, however, is not the same as a conceptual focus. Holism refers to how the nurse uses the concepts to approach a patient, family, or community health situation. Holism involves the use of multiple concepts to address the many factors and challenges that are present in any encounter. Holism thus provides a perspective or framework for ensuring that multiple concepts are addressed in the situation as appropriate. A conceptual focus emphasizes the concepts and knowledge that are used to create that holistic approach.

Summary

As the health care environment becomes increasingly complex, nursing programs need to respond by preparing graduates to manage information effectively, provide patient-centered care that is evidence based, and work well within teams. This requires a transformation of nursing education curricula and teaching practices from an instructor-centered and content-focused paradigm to the conceptual approach. This chapter introduces the conceptual approach, reinforcing the notion that six key elements—concepts, exemplars, concept-based curriculum, concept-based instruction, conceptual learning, and evaluation of learning—must be in place for optimal success (see Box 1.1). Benefits of the conceptual approach include addressing content saturation, information management, enhanced student learning and engagement, collaboration, and supporting the development of clinical judgment. In the chapters that follow, key elements and processes are presented in greater detail to enhance understanding and application in teaching practice.

References

Alfayoumi I. The impact of combining concept-based learning and concept-mapping pedagogies on nursing students' clinical reasoning abilities. *Nurse Educ Today.* 2019;72:40–46.

Alligood MR. *Nursing Theorists and Their Work.* 10th ed. St. Louis, MO: Elsevier; 2022.

Ambrose SA, Bridges MW, DiPietro M, et al. *How Learning Works. 7 Research-Based Principles for Smart Teaching.* San Francisco, CA: Jossey-Bass; 2010.

Bellack J. Letting go of the rock. *J Nurs Educ.* 2008;47(10):439–440.

Bransford JD, Brown AL, Cocking RR. *How People Learn: Brain, Mind, Experience, and School.* Washington, DC: National Academy Press; 2000.

Carrieri-Kohlman V, Lindsey AM, West CM. *Pathophysiological Phenomena in Nursing: Human Response to Illness.* 3rd ed. Philadelphia, PA: Saunders; 2003.

Deane W, Asselin M. Transitioning to concept-based teaching: a discussion of strategies and the use of Bridge's change model. *J Nurs Educ Pract.* 2015;5(10):52–59.

Diekelmann N. "Too much content…." Epistemologies' grasp and nursing education. *J Nurs Educ.* 2002;41(11):469–470.

Diekelmann N, Smythe E. Teacher talk: new pedagogies for nursing. Covering the content and the additive curriculum: how can I use my time with students to best help them learn what they need to know. *J Nurs Educ.* 2004;43(8):341–344.

Erikson L. *Concept-Based Curriculum and Instruction.* Thousand Oaks, CA: Corwin Press; 2002.

Erikson L. *Stirring the Head, Heart, and Soul. Redefining Curriculum, Instruction, and Concept-Based Learning.* Thousand Oaks, CA: Corwin Press; 2008.

Erickson L, Lanning LA, French R. *Concept-Based Curriculum and Instruction for the Thinking Classroom.* Thousand Oaks, CA: Corwin Press; 2017.

Forbes MO, Hickey MT. Curriculum reform in baccalaureate nursing education: review of the literature. *Int J Nurs Educ Schol.* 2009;6(1):Article 27.

Giddens J, Brady D. Rescuing nursing education from content saturation: the case for a concept-based curriculum. *J Nurs Educ.* 2007;46(2):65–69.

Giddens J, Brady D, Brown P, et al. A new curriculum for a new era of nursing education. *Nurs Educ Perspect.* 2008;29(4):200–204.

Gonzalez L. Teaching clinical reasoning piece by piece: a clinical reasoning concept-based learning method. *J Nurs Educ.* 2018;57(12):727–735.

Hendricks SM, Wangerin V. Concept-based curriculum: changing attitudes and overcoming barriers. *Nurs Educ.* 2017;42(3):138–142.

Interprofessional Education Collaborative Expert Panel. *Core Competencies for Interprofessional Collaborative Practice: Report of an Expert Panel.* Washington, DC: Interprofessional Education Collaborative; 2011.

Ironside PM. "Covering content" and teaching thinking: deconstructing the additive curriculum. *J Nurs Educ.* 2004;43(1):5–12.

Lasater K, Nielsen A. The influence on concept-based learning activities on students' clinical judgement development. *J Nurs Edu.* 2009;48(8):441–446.

Lucey CR. Achieving Competency-Based, Time Variable Health Professions Education. In: *Proceeding of a conference sponsored by Josiah Macy Jr. Foundation in June 2017. Macy Jr. Foundation;* 2018.

National League for Nursing. Position Statement: Innovation in Nursing Education. *A Call to Reform.* 2003. http://www.nln.org/docs/default-source/about/archived-position-statements/innovation-in-nursing-education-a-call-to-reform-pdf.pdf?sfvrsn=4.

Nielsen A. Concept-based learning activities using the clinical judgement model as a foundation for clinical learning. *J Nurs Educ.* 2009;48(6):350–354.

Nielsen A. Concept-based learning in clinical experiences: brining theory to clinical education for deep learning. *J Nurs Educ.* 2016;55(7):365–371.

Orem D, *Nursing Concepts of Practice.* Columbus, OH: McGraw-Hill; 1971.

Quality and Safety Education for Nurses Institute. *Competencies.* n.d. http://qsen.org/competencies/.

Royal KD, Zakrajsek T. Good teaching is not a race to cover content: less can be more. *Ear Nose Throat J.* 2017;96:402–404.

Rodgers B. Concepts, analysis, and the development of nursing knowledge: the evolutionary cycle. *J Adv Nurs.* 1989;14:330–335.

Rosch E. Reclaiming concepts. *J Conscious Stud.* 1999;6:61–78.

Schmidt WH, McKnight CC, Raizen S. In: *A Splintered Vision: An Investigation of U.S. Science and Mathematics Education. U.S. National Research Center for the Third International Mathematics and Science Study (TIMSS).* Dordrecht, Netherlands: Kluwer Academic Publishers; 1997.

Sousa DA. *Mind, Brain, and Education. Neuroscience Implications for the Classroom.* Bloomington, IN: Solution Tree Press; 2010.

Taba H. *Teaching Strategies and Cognitive Functioning in Elementary School Children. Cooperative Research Project.* Washington, DC: Office of Education, U.S. Department of Health, Education, and Welfare; 1966.

Tanner CA. Thinking like a nurse: a research-based model of clinical judgment in nursing. *J Nurs Educ.* 2006;45(6):204–211.

Timpson WM, Bendel-Simso P. *Concepts and Choices for Teaching: Meeting the Challenges in Higher Education.* Madison, WI: Magna Publications; 1996.

CHAPTER 2

Differentiating Concept-Based and Competency-Based Approaches

A growing trend in higher education has been the use of competencies as a framework for education and evaluation of student learning. In a competency-based approach, students are expected to demonstrate key behaviors and activities that are considered critical for a defined area. Performance expectations are made explicit to learners; faculty ensure students have multiple opportunities for learning and demonstration of the competencies in multiple situations.

With continued and growing issues in health care delivery, the state of health professions education has come into question. The delivery of high-quality health care requires a workforce that is optimally prepared to practice in an increasingly complex system. Thus, calls for radical transformation of all health professions education have occurred, with an eye toward transitioning to a competency-based approach (Lucey, 2018). This need has been further fueled by the steady decline in initial competency of new graduate registered nurses over the past 15 years (Kavanagh and Sharpnack, 2021).

The competency-based approach for education and evaluation has been present in the health professions literature and in the general education literature for years. Widespread adoption has been slow due to a lack of widely accepted definitions of what constitutes an individual competency and the wide variability in terms of scope and measurability of competencies that have been developed. Regardless, competency-based education will continue to evolve as competencies needed for quality care delivery are further defined and clarified.

Many professional organizations in the health professions have adopted or are in the process of adopting this method. The American Association of Medical Education adopted a competency-based framework for medical education, influenced by the work of Englander et al. (2013). Other health care disciplines including pharmacy and dentistry have engaged in the identification and creation of core competencies for their respective professions (Commission on Dental Accreditation, n.d.; McLaughlin et al., 2017). Nursing has also engaged in discussions regarding competency-based education, leading to the adoption of a competency-based approach for nursing education by the American Association of Colleges of Nursing (AACN), as reflected in *The Essentials: Core Competencies for Professional Nursing Education* (AACN, 2021).

Those familiar with concept-based education may wonder how competency-based education fits within a concept-based model. What is the difference between a concept and a domain? What is the difference between a concept and a competency? What is the difference between a competence and a competency? The purpose of this chapter is to clarify these distinctions, show the interrelated nature of concept-based and competency-based approaches, and clarify how these approaches complement and enhance one another.

Defining Competence, Competency, and Competency-Based Education

Noted earlier, one of the challenges associated with a competency-based approach has been the lack of a universal definition or understandings of competence and competency.

Competence is a term that reflects an individual's ability to do something successfully. It is a term that often is used to describe a person's ability in a wide variety of ways. The related term *competent* is used as an adjective to describe a person who possesses expected skill, ability, and/or qualifications (e.g., a competent driver, a competent teacher, a competent nurse). The term *incompetent* is used as a negative reference to one who lacks required abilities or who has failed to perform at a level expected (an incompetent carpenter, as an example).

A useful definition of competence offered by Frank, Snell, and colleagues is "The array of abilities (knowledge, skills, attitudes) across multiple domains or aspects of performance in a certain context. Competency is multidimensional and dynamic. It changes with time, experience, and settings" (Frank et al., 2010, p. 641). The American Nurses Association (ANA) describes competence as an individual performing at an expected level (ANA, 2021).

Similarly, definitions of competency incorporate abilities (knowledge, skills, attitudes), with key distinctions associated with the expectation of a learner and that the competency is observable and measurable. As described by Frank and colleagues, competency is *"An observable ability of a health professional, integrating multiple components such as knowledge, skills, and attitudes. Since competencies are observable, they can be measured and assessed to ensure their acquisition"* (Frank et al., 2010, p. 641). A similar definition of competency, as proposed by Englander and colleagues, is *"An observable ability of a health care professional, integrating multiple components such as knowledge, skills, and attitudes"* (Englander et al., 2013, p. 1089). The ANA's definition of competency is similar yet slightly different: *"an expected level of performance that integrates knowledge, skills, abilities, and judgment"* (ANA, 2021, p. 52).

It should be of no surprise that a definition of competency-based education builds on the idea of providing learning experiences framed around defined competencies that support the development of competence. As it relates to medical education, Frank and colleagues defined competency-based medical education as *"An outcomes-based approach to the design, implementation, assessment, and evaluation of medical education programs, using an organizing framework of competencies."* (Frank et al., 2010, p. 641). In the K-12 literature, competency-based education is described in a learner-centric paradigm whereby students are empowered to make *"decisions about their learning experiences, how they will create and apply knowledge, and how they will demonstrate their learning"* (Levine and Patrick, 2019, p. 3). In the general education paradigm, competency-based education incorporates ideas including student empowerment regarding their learning, assessment, supporting individual needs of learners, varied pace of learning, and rigorous common expectations for learning (Levine and Patrick, 2019). Comparisons of definitions among the various terms is presented in Box 2.1.

Competency-based education requires an intentional identification of specific competencies expected of learners, a plan for ensuring learners have multiple experiences to learn the competencies in a variety of situations and varying complexity with ongoing feedback, and that there are clear and consistent ways to observe and assess that learning. Perhaps one of the most important benefits of a competency-based approach is that the expectations of what learners should be able to do with what they know is explicit and these expectations are built around what is expected of a competent practitioner. For this reason, the use of competencies is particularly important as a foundation for clinical education.

BOX 2.1 ■ Definitions

Competence:
- The array of abilities (knowledge, skills, attitudes) across multiple domains or aspects of performance in a certain context. Competency is multidimensional and dynamic. It changes with time, experience, and settings (Frank et al., 2010, p. 641).
- An individual performing at an expected level (ANA, 2021, p. 52)

Competency:
- An observable ability of a health professional, integrating multiple components such as knowledge, skills, and attitudes. Since competencies are observable, they can be measured and assessed to ensure their acquisition (Frank et al., 2010, p. 641).
- An observable ability of a health care professional, integrating multiple components such as knowledge, skills, and attitudes (Englander et al., 2013, p. 1089).
- An expected level of performance that integrates knowledge, skills, abilities, and judgment (ANA, 2021, p. 52)

Competency-Based Education:
- An outcomes-based approach to the design, implementation, assessment, and evaluation of medical education programs, using an organizing framework of competencies (Frank et al., 2010, p. 641).
- Students are empowered to make "decisions about their learning experiences, how they will create and apply knowledge, and how they will demonstrate their learning" (Levine and Patrick, 2019, p. 3).

Origins and Progression of the Competency-Based Approach

An emphasis on competencies in education is not new. One could argue that it has evolved out of the outcomes-based education movement. Early in the 20th century, traditional curriculum development, reflected by the work of Tyler (1949), focused on program goals and objectives organized around instructional or knowledge-based objectives. An emphasis on instructional objectives (which focus on things an instructor intends to teach) subsequently led to a greater emphasis on the educational process as opposed to the educational end-product. Outcome-based education arose as an alternative perspective, with an emphasis in program and learner outcomes, as opposed to the instructional process to attain them. Learning outcomes (often referred to as student learning outcomes, or SLOs) are statements of what students will achieve as a result of the learning process. From this perspective, the desired curriculum outcomes drive curriculum decisions; curriculum processes (including instruction) are secondary (Rubin and Spady, 1984).

Competency-based education is a type of outcome-based education, with clearly defined competencies used to delineate the outcomes of learning. Calls for competency-based approaches have appeared in the literature across multiple professions and disciplines for decades. In the 1970s, Del Bueno described competency-based nursing education from two perspectives: as a broad concept used as the conceptual framework for a curriculum, or as the framework for units of instruction such as a learning module (Del Bueno, 1978). In either perspective, Del Bueno emphasized the focus was on learning outcomes. As competency-based education models have matured, the application of competencies has focused on program outcomes as opposed to individual learning modules.

Today, competency statements in health sciences describe the behaviors and skills expected of graduates. Demonstration of competency achievement occurs in many instances over time as opposed to a single point in time in an isolated course. Table 2.1 presents examples of three competency statements proposed by Englander and colleagues that reflect physician competencies.

TABLE 2.1 ■ **Examples of Physician Competency Statements**

Domain	Competency Statement
Interpersonal and Communication Skills	"Communicate effectively with patients, families, and the public, as appropriate across a broad range of socioeconomic and cultural backgrounds."
Systems-Based Practice	"Coordinate patient care within the health care system relevant to one's clinical specialty."
Personal and Professional Development	"Provide leadership skills that enhance team functioning, the learning environment, and/or the health care delivery system."

From Englander R, Cameron T, Ballar AJ, et al. Toward a taxonomy of competency domains for health professions and competencies for physicians. *Acad Med.* 2013;88(8):1088–1094.

Contemporary competency-based education in health education is grounded in the philosophy that education should be designed with an "explicit and relentless focus on the needs of patients and society for improved health and healthcare" (Lucey, 2018). Such a focus requires adaptability in the curriculum development and implementation process. The competency-based approach supports the diverse learning goals and needs of students, acknowledging that students can guide their own learning. Furthermore, because of the diverse learning needs of learners, the amount of time needed to demonstrate the competencies varies, meaning a student might need less time or more time to demonstrate competence compared to other students.

MISCONCEPTIONS AND CLARIFICATIONS

Misconception: Competency-based education is a new and innovative idea.	*Clarification:* Competency-based education has been present in the literature for over 50 years. Thus, competency-based education is not a new idea, but rather an idea that has gained in clarity and prominence.

Working toward a competency-based, time-variable approach in health professions education is a specific recommendation from a panel of experts who came together to discuss the issues in health professions education. A few examples of successful competency-based, time-variable programs in the health sciences exist. As one example, the University of Wisconsin currently supports a flexible option for Bachelor of Science in nursing degree completion using this model (Litwack and Brower, 2018). A time-variable approach such as this represents a disruption to higher education; enacting such an approach on a large scale will be challenging due to the long-standing traditional views of higher education held by faculty and administrators, structural constraints within higher education, licensing requirements, and accreditation standards (Lucey, 2018). Despite these challenges, there is momentum among leaders across disciplines for time variability in competency-based education, thus this may evolve in the future.

Intersection of Concepts and Competencies: How Do These Approaches Fit?

The information regarding competencies and competency-based education in the previous sections provided helpful background to understand the topic. However, for the purposes of this chapter and this book, the incorporation of competencies and the evaluation of competencies are discussed in the context of the conceptual approach.

The application of competencies within the conceptual approach requires a clear understanding of the terms used in competency-based education and how these are different than, and similar to, terms used in concept-based approaches. Specifically, clarity is needed regarding differences and similarities between:

- concept and domain
- concept and competency

More importantly, by gaining an understanding of these distinctions one will see that domains, concepts, and competencies are complementary in nature, and serve as enhancements to learning as opposed to competing ideas.

WHAT IS THE DIFFERENCE BETWEEN A CONCEPT AND A DOMAIN?

In the competency-based education literature, domains are, by design, the organizational units for competencies. A domain is a grouping of similar elements, providing an overarching structure or framework. Likewise, in a concept-based approach, concepts represent an organizing idea or mental construct that serves as the overarching structure or framework of information associated with the concept. Put another way, concepts and domains represent broad ideas and principles that are useful frameworks to provide structure for learning. An umbrella serves as a useful cognitive image to illustrate and remember this point (Fig. 2.1). So, is there a difference? The primary distinction is that the term "domain" tends to be directly linked to competency statements. They both represent organizing ideas and principles, they both provide a framework for curriculum design, they both provide a structure for learning, and competencies can be used as outcome statements for learning in both paradigms—thus, concepts and domains are really more similar than different (Box 2.2).

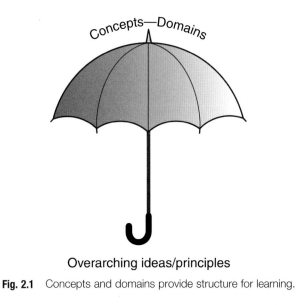

Concepts—Domains

Overarching ideas/principles

Fig. 2.1 Concepts and domains provide structure for learning.

> **BOX 2.2 ▨ Commonalities Between Domains and Concepts**
>
> - Represent organizing ideas and principles
> - Used as a framework for curriculum design
> - Provide structure for learning
> - Are evaluated through competency assessment

WHAT IS THE DIFFERENCE BETWEEN A CONCEPT AND A COMPETENCY?

In the previous section, the similarities between concepts and domains were established. Next, it is helpful to gain an appreciation for differences and similarities in competencies and concepts. Various definitions of competence and competencies were presented earlier in the chapter. At face value, and if just considering definitions, the terms *concept* and *competency* clearly are different. A concept is an overarching idea, grounded in research and reflects an area of core disciplinary knowledge, whereas a competency is a statement describing what is expected to competently carry out a function. Competencies are presented from the perspective of Knowledge, Skills, and Abilities (or Attitudes)—referred to as KSAs. The competency statement is explicit, observable, and measurable; an individual must integrate the KSAs to effectively demonstrate a competency. Thus, the primary distinction between these two terms is that a concept represents a broad idea or principle whereas a competency is a specific statement of expected performance as it relates to the concept.

MISCONCEPTIONS AND CLARIFICATIONS

Misconception: Competencies and concepts are pretty much the same.	***Clarification:*** Concepts and competencies are different, yet complementary in nature. A concept represents an overarching idea, or a broad area of knowledge. A competency is a statement of what a person should be able to do—in other words, a performance expectation. Competencies are often used as a method for outcomes measurement of a broader concept.

COMPLEMENTARY RELATIONSHIP BETWEEN CONCEPTS AND COMPETENCIES IN EDUCATION

Although concepts and competencies are clearly not the same, they have a complementary relationship from an educational context. The outcome of conceptual learning involves gaining knowledge and skills associated with the concept, and the ability to apply knowledge and skills in a variety of contexts. In the case of nursing education, the application occurs within the context of patient care (Fig. 2.2). A strong cognitive understanding and skill base is needed to support

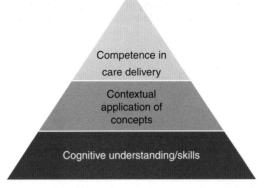

Fig. 2.2 Teaching conceptually leads to competency attainment in the clinical setting.

assessment, clinical decisions, and professional actions in the delivery of nursing care. In her landmark work *Teaching in Nursing*, Benner and colleagues called for a shift from a focus covering decontextualized knowledge, to an emphasis on teaching for a sense of salience, situational cognition, and an application in particular situations (Benner et al., 2010). This is truly at the heart of concept-based instruction.

Concept-based instruction uses concepts to guide teaching and learning. Students organize their thinking around concepts. Conceptual teaching strategies intentionally facilitate conceptual learning by helping learners link new information or information in a different context to things previously learned through cognitive connections. Over time, the learner gains an increasingly sophisticated ability to apply that information in a number of contexts. The rapid and continuous advances in health care require that graduates are skilled in conceptual thinking and clinical reasoning to adapt to these changes.

Competencies naturally complement conceptual learning through robust assessment. When competencies are associated with a concept, expectations are clear for both students and faculty. Because competencies are intentionally written in observable and measurable terms, they provide valid and reliable ways to assess learning through demonstrated performance that requires the integration of knowledge, skills, values, and beliefs. Competency assessment occurs over time, in multiple situations.

Therefore, where concepts represent the structural organization of knowledge to be learned, competencies provide the structure and process for performance and evaluation. Table 2.2 shows the complementary intent of concepts and competencies. Concept-based learning requires the application of concept knowledge and skills as part of the learning experience in a "real-world" context. Conceptual learning is evaluated using competency assessment in that competencies describe the intended outcome, not the learning process (Giddens, 2020). As an outcome statement, a competency can be applied to any learning activity, learning module, course, or curriculum. The true opportunity lies in the application of competencies as a robust process for outcome measurement in a concept-based curriculum.

TABLE 2.2 ■ **Concepts and Competencies in Education**

Concept-Based Learning	Competency Assessment
Focus on overarching principle or ideas with emphasis in: • Knowledge and skill acquisition • Application in clinical context • Appropriate actions in clinical care	The observable performance of the learner through the integration of: • Knowledge • Skills • Attitudes/Abilities

LINKAGES BETWEEN CONCEPT-BASED CURRICULA AND COMPETENCY-BASED EDUCATION IN NURSING

Earlier in this chapter, it was established that competencies and domains are very similar. It should be no surprise then that many of the concepts typically found in concept-based curricula are similar to, or the same as, the domains common to competency-based education. To illustrate this point, Table 2.3 presents a cross-walk comparing common nursing concepts to common domains of competence for health care. As can be seen, there is variability in the titles used or the combination of ideas under a title, but the concepts and domains essentially represent similar ideas. To take this a step further, AACN identified eight *featured* concepts (clinical judgment; communication; compassionate care; diversity, equity, and inclusion; ethics; evidence-based practice; health policy; and social determinates of health) within the *Essentials,* noting that these concepts are "interrelated and interwoven within the domains and competencies" (AACN, 2021, p.12). Many of the AACN concepts are those also found in a concept-based curriculum and are also consistent with domains identified by other organizations.

Concepts are also often categorically grouped by like-concepts. Three common concept groupings that are discussed in Chapter 4 include:

- Health Care Recipient Concepts (such as development, functional ability, family dynamics);
- Health and Illness Concepts (such as perfusion, gas exchange, infection, cognition);
- Professional Nursing and Health Care Concepts (such as collaboration, leadership, ethics, health care quality).

One might notice that the domains used for the competency-based approach closely align with the Professional Nursing and Health Care Concepts category. Concepts in this category describe the behaviors and context of care of the nurse practicing in health care. These are consistent with the same domains and competencies that focus on what the health professionals will do—in other words, the specific actions and outcomes that are linked to the domains and related competencies.

One domain of competence centers around the care of patients—such as Person-Centered Care (as identified by AACN); Patient-Centered Care (identified by QSEN); Patient Care (identified by Englander); and Standards of Practice (identified by the ANA). This type of domain represents competencies associated

TABLE 2.3 ■ **Nursing Concepts and Related Domains of Competence**

Nursing Concept	Competency Domains
Collaboration	• Interprofessional Partnerships (AACN) • Interprofessional Collaboration (Englander) • Teamwork and Team-Based Practice (IPEC) • Teamwork and Collaboration (QSEN) • Collaboration (ANA)
Communication	• Interpersonal and Communication Practices (IPEC) • Communication (ANA) • Interpersonal and Communication Skills (Englander)
Professionalism	• Professionalism (AACN) • Professionalism (Englander) • Professional Practice Evaluation (ANA)
Leadership	• Personal, Professional, and Leadership Development (AACN) • Personal and Professional Development (Englander et al., 2013) • Leadership (ANA)
Health Care Organizations; Health Systems	• Systems-based practice (Englander) • Systems-based practice (AACN)
Quality; Safety	• Quality and Safety (AACN) • Practice-based learning and improvement (Englander) • Safety (QSEN) • Quality Improvement (QSEN) • Quality of Practice (ANA)
Technology and Informatics	• Informatics and Health Care Technology (AACN) • Informatics (QSEN)

Note: *AACN*, American Association of Colleges of Nursing. *The Essentials: Core Competencies for Professional Nursing Education*. Washington, DC: AACN; 2021; *ANA*, American Nurses Association. *Scope and Standards of Practice*. 4th ed. Silver Spring, MD: ANA; 2021; *Englander*, Englander R, Cameron T, Ballar AJ, et al. Toward a taxonomy of competency domains for health professions and competencies for physicians. *Acad Med*. 2013;88(8):1088–1094; *IPEC*, Interprofessional Education Collaborative, https://www.ipecollaborative.org/; *QSEN*, Quality and Safety Education for Nurses, https://qsen.org/.

with the delivery of care to a patient. This domain is broader than others because the competencies reflect general activities (taking a history, conducting a health assessment, diagnosing health problems, developing a plan of care, implementing interventions for that care, and evaluating patient outcomes) across the age continuum, across the care continuum, and across health conditions. It is intended that these activities are applied in all settings as appropriate, but the specific knowledge and skills about the various health conditions encountered in practice is not represented within these competencies.

In a concept-based nursing curriculum, multiple concepts related to patient care are used for the development of conceptual understandings related to health conditions of patients. Such concepts (such as gas exchange, nutrition, mobility, perfusion, cognition, stress and coping, and cellular regulation) ensure students gain knowledge, skill, and clinical judgment around foundational care concepts linked to health conditions they will encounter in clinical practice. The broader patient care concepts found under domains of person-centered care still apply; it is just that the concepts provide clarity regarding the specific application of these competencies within the concept. For example, when students learn about the concept of gas exchange the associated knowledge and skills needed to provide care (conducting an assessment, plan care, provide appropriate care interventions) are discussed in the context of gas exchange, so that the student can support a person to optimize gas exchange. In other words, the competencies of "Patient Care" are applied within specific contexts, based on the need of the patient. A student ultimately demonstrates competence in a domain such as patient-centered care through interventions in multiple patient situations and contexts, and most importantly demonstrating the ability to transfer learning from one situation to another. This is at the heart of both concept-based and competency-based approaches. Because of this interrelationship, we do not differentiate "teaching" the concept and competency—the practical difference is the techniques and methods used to evaluate student learning.

Summary

The structure of a concept-based curriculum lends itself well to the use and application of competencies. Stated previously, competencies are organized within a domain or concept and each domain/concept has multiple competencies. Nursing schools with a concept-based curricula can use concepts to organize competency statements to guide the expected outcomes and assessment for learners. The desired learning outcome of conceptual learning is that the student will know what the concept is, recognize the concept in clinical practice, and know what to do about it. This closely aligns with the idea that competencies articulate the expectation of what a learner can do with what they know.

The interrelationships between concepts, domains, and competencies are discussed throughout this book. In Chapter 3, there is a discussion regarding how to incorporate competencies within a concept presentation. In Chapter 4, the incorporation of competencies in concept-based curricula and program assessment is discussed. In Chapter 8 the use of competencies is incorporated into the discussion regarding the evaluation of student learning.

The concept-based and competency-based approaches in education are interrelated and should not be perceived as competing ideas. Concepts are useful for creating a framework for the curriculum and the competencies provide clear expectations; these are complementary in nature (Giddens, 2020). Nursing faculty will find that a concept-based curriculum aligns well with the incorporation of competencies. Additional discussion regarding competency integration within a concept-based curriculum can be found in the chapters that follow.

References

American Association of Colleges of Nursing. *The Essentials: Core Competencies for Professional Nursing Education.* Washington, DC: AACN; 2021.

American Nurses Association. *Nursing: Scope and Standards of Practice.* 4th ed. Silver Spring, MD: ANA; 2021.

Benner P, Sutphen M, Leonard V, et al. *Educating Nurses: A Call for Radical Transformation.* San Francisco, CA: Josey-Bass; 2010.

Commission on Dental Accreditation (n.d.). *Standards for Predoctoral Dental Education.* https://www.ada.org/en/coda/current-accreditation-standards.

Del Bueno DJ. Competency based education. *Nurse Educ.* 1978;3(3):10–14.

Englander R, Cameron T, Ballar AJ, et al. Toward a taxonomy of competency domains for health professions and competencies for physicians. *Acad Med.* 2013;88(8):1088–1094. https://doi.org/10.1097/ACM.0b013e31829a3b2b.

Frank JR, Snell LS, Cate OT, et al. Competency-based medical education: theory to practice. *Med Teach.* 2010;32(8):638–645. https://doi.org/10.3109/0142159X.2010.501190.

Giddens JL. Demystifying concept-based and competency-based approaches. *J Nurs Educ.* 2020;59(3):123–124. https://doi.org/10.3928/01484834-20200220-01.

Kavanagh J, Sharpnack P. Crisis in competency: a defining moment for nursing education. *Online J Issues Nurs.* 2021;26(1).

Levine E, Patrick S. *What is Competency-Based Education: An Updated Definition.* Aurora Institute: Vienna, VA; 2019.

Litwack K, Brower AM. The University of Wisconsin-Milwaukee flexible option for bachelor of science in nursing degree completion. *Acad Med.* 2018;93(3):S37–S41. https://doi.org/10.1097/ACM.0000000000002076.

Lucey CR. Achieving Competency-Based Time-Variable Health Professions Education. In: *Proceedings of a conference sponsored by Josiah Macy Jr. Foundation in June 2017; New York, NY;* 2018. https://macyfoundation.org/assets/reports/publications/macy_monograph_2017_final.pdf.

McLaughlin JE, Bush AA, Rodgers PT, et al. Exploring the requisite skills and competencies of pharmacists needed for success in an evolving health care environment. *Am J Pharm Educ.* 2017;81(6):116. https://doi.org/10.5688/ajpe816116.

Rubin SE, Spady WG. Achieving excellence through outcome-based instructional delivery. *Educ Leadership.* 1984;41(8):37–44.

Tyler RW. *Basic Principles of Curriculum and Instruction.* Chicago, IL: University of Chicago Press; 1949.

CHAPTER 3

Concepts for the Nursing Discipline

Successful adoption of the conceptual approach in nursing requires that a conceptual foundation for nursing be at the forefront of teaching and learning. In traditional approaches to teaching, facts and examples receive most of the attention, with thinking about those facts and examples occurring on a more abstract level. In the conceptual approach, thinking takes center stage. For this approach to be successful, faculty must have a thorough understanding of concepts, including what they are, how they are formed, how they represent the discipline of nursing, and what functions they serve regarding knowledge overall.

In addition to having a clear idea about what concepts are in general, faculty need to have a shared understanding and agreement about the concepts used in a curriculum, so students are not confused by faculty members offering different or even opposing interpretations. This chapter provides an overview of concepts, clarification of concepts within the nursing discipline, and the development of concepts for consistent use within a curriculum. Attempts to implement a conceptual approach cannot be successful if faculty lack a strong foundation as it relates to understanding concepts.

An Overview of Concepts

WHAT IS A CONCEPT?

A thorough discussion of concepts can go in numerous directions because concepts have many roles in human existence. In the simplest of terms, humans organize thinking and ideas around concepts; thus, a concept is a mental or cognitive organization. Concepts are major components of knowledge, theoretical constructions, and organizational tools for thinking. They also can be creative elements, ideas or mental images, essential components of communication, and parts of larger theories. All of these foci point not only to the critical nature of concepts in human cognition and learning but also to the many different roles and uses of concepts that need to be considered to develop a clear understanding of what a concept is.

From a knowledge standpoint, a concept is "an abstraction that is expressed in some form" (Rodgers, 1989, p. 332). This may seem like a rather simple statement to reflect the essential nature of concepts and the many roles that they play in human existence. Yet this idea of being abstract and being linked to some form of expression is at the core of the definition of a concept. In general, concepts are formed in the mind as people encounter different situations and begin to see similarities in those encounters. As a result of these experiences, the mind forms images that include common characteristics and the person also learns what word goes along with those images.

A child learning what is meant by the word "dog" is a simple example of this process. The child might live with a retriever, visit a family that has a terrier, and have a neighbor with a poodle. The child will hear the word "dog" used to refer to those animals. In a short amount of time the child recognizes that these creatures have some things in common and that the word "dog" does not refer to any specific animal but is applicable to an array of animals that have certain characteristics in common. Hearing the word "dog" stimulates a mental image or idea—that is, the concept of *Dog* that has been formed from a composite of those common characteristics. "Max" would be an example of a proper name for a specific dog; "dog" is the term used to express an idea of general characteristics common to all dogs. In conversation, someone might say, "I have a dog," and the person to whom he or she is speaking will immediately know something about the animal to which the original speaker is referring even if that animal is not present during the conversation. The concept that is stimulated on hearing the word "dog" does not specify the type of dog, age, size, or activity level; rather, each individual may have a distinct concept of *Dog* based on experience, familiarity, exposure, and even preference. In spite of individual variation in interpretation, however, everyone involved will be able to converse about these creatures because each has a functional concept of *Dog*. This example shows how the grasping of a concept, based on recognition of common characteristics, makes it possible to refer to something that is not present, to understand such references, and to understand each other and have meaningful communication (Rodgers, 2000). It is also evident, based on this example, how learning, or developing a grasp of particular concepts, makes it possible to carry that concept to different situations and conversations and perhaps to new encounters with different dogs. Without the ability to organize thoughts and ideas into concepts, it would not be possible to navigate the world, to communicate about it, or to make good decisions about actions.

Concepts are acquired in different ways, but, as the previous example indicates, socialization can be an important part of the process. If the child is only exposed to small dogs, the concept will be constructed on the basis of that exposure and familiarity. The child who later encounters a Great Dane or Mastiff might find that his or her initial concept of *Dog* is challenged and will have to reevaluate, or learn in a new way, that these situations are also appropriate for application of the concept of *Dog*. This has important implications for a conceptual approach to teaching—that is, bringing attention to the way in which the students are exposed to examples of various concepts and the array of variations in application.

A person forms an understanding of concepts in other ways because not all concepts have physical examples to facilitate their learning. Concepts such as *Ethics, Grief, Safety,* and *Leadership* are very important in nursing, but do not have corresponding physical objects that can be pointed to as examples of these concepts. In such instances the abstract nature of concepts should be obvious. Such concepts are developed through exposure to ideas, human creativity, storytelling, and experiencing situations in which the concept exists, even if those situations are not specifically related to the concept on a one-to-one basis, as is the case with physical objects. These examples also make it easy to see how socialization, education, personal experience, and values can influence the particular concept that any nurse holds. Cultural differences in the expression of and norms surrounding many of these concepts are documented extensively. *Grief* is a particularly good example of how norms vary in the formation of a concept (Cowles and Rodgers, 2000), and the value and expressions of autonomy vary with age, gender, and other demographic factors.

MISCONCEPTIONS AND CLARIFICATIONS

Misconception: A concept is something that can be seen or directly measured.	**Clarification:** Although some concepts can be represented by a physical object, many concepts do not have a corresponding physical object and are represented by ideas, abstractions, mental images, or other modalities.

PHILOSOPHICAL VIEWS OF CONCEPTS

Concepts are found throughout a large volume of literature in numerous disciplines. Sociologists have discussed concepts as indicators of societies and group behavior, in addition to the role of concepts and conceptual problems in their own discipline (Lizardo, 2013; Sundbo, 2013); anthropologists have undertaken similar work in areas related to culture and acculturation. Cognitive psychologists rely on an understanding of concepts in explanations of learning and knowledge acquisition (Mahon and Caramazza, 2009). Educators across multiple disciplines also use concepts as a basis for teaching, learning, and knowledge acquisition (Ambrose et al., 2010; Erickson et al., 2017; Renkl, 2017; Timpson and Bendel-Simso, 1996).

There are two major traditions in the discussion of concepts: the *entity view* and the *dispositional view*. Each of these views has a unique philosophical perspective regarding what concepts are, how they are formed, and what purpose they serve relative to the external world.

Entity View of Concepts

In simple terms, an entity view considers concepts to be *things* (entities). Consistent with most philosophers who espouse such a view, these things are *ideas* in the mind. Concepts are objects or specific things that can be examined and evaluated on their own; and external references exist against which concepts can be judged. In other words, according to an entity view, concepts exist in the mind as objects of thinking, and these concepts relate to examples that can be found in physical reality. Furthermore, there is a strict interpretation of the definition of the concept and the attributes that constitute the definition of the concept. The attributes are clustered together to capture characteristics that are common in similar objects or occurrences. From the perspective of the entity view, evaluation of whether or not someone has a grasp of the concept is focused on exploring that actual concept—the definition, rules, and conditions that make up the concept.

Dispositional View of Concepts

Presenting a contrast to the entity view are dispositional theories of concepts. In a dispositional view, concepts are abstractions, not things themselves; a concept is regarded as a behavior or, more specifically, a capability for a particular behavior. It is not enough to just be able to list the concept attributes. The person who understands the concept also can act on that knowledge in a way that is appropriate to show an accurate or functional understanding. From a dispositional view, evaluation of learning aligns well with competency-based assessment. The relationship between concepts and competencies is discussed in Chapter 2.

Application of Entity and Dispositional Views in Education

Both views are useful and should not be a considered as "right or wrong" or "better or worse"— rather, the different ways concepts may be approached. Specifically, faculty should be aware that both views have value in teaching. That said, some concepts more logically align with one view over another. As one example, the concept of *Health* is easier to approach from a dispositional view than an entity view. *Health* is not a single object; rather, it is something that can be present in varying degrees and in widely different ways in different people and contexts. Health is something that tends to exist "more or less." There is no single thing that goes by the name "health" that could match a concept of *Health* as needed in an entity view. Although it may be possible to identify, or at least construct a single outstanding example of *Health*, being able to say about a particular instance "this is health" and "this is not health" is not realistic and does not represent a practical application.

Regardless of the focus used, concepts constitute an important component of knowledge, learning, socialization, and human existence. Conceptual learning requires a focus on knowledge before action; the acquisition of cognitive content enables more widespread application than a focus on specific tasks or activities would allow. Table 3.1 presents a comparison of entity view and dispositional views of concepts and Box 3.1 presents an example of one concept framed both ways.

TABLE 3.1 ■ A Comparison of Entity and Dispositional Views of Concepts

In Entity Views, the Concept	In Dispositional Views, the Concept
• Is composed of necessary and sufficient conditions that are absolute (Essentialism)	• Is composed of attributes that may be fluid or fuzzy (Probabilism)
• Has clear boundaries	• May show some variation across contexts
• Adheres to strict rules of use	• Examples have some features in common but may not be identical
• Corresponds with an actual object or thing	
• Is associated with a distinct idea or mental image that enables labeling and categorization	• Is associated with a mental image that may enable certain competencies related to the concept
• Corresponds to real objects that share the same features	• Exemplars serve as prototypes rather than absolutes
• Corresponds to a particular word	• May be expressed using different words

---

BOX 3.1 ■ A Conceptual Exemplar of Entity and Dispositional Views

Concept: DOG

Entity view: The individual has a solid understanding of the definition, attributes, and correctly identifying a dog.

Dispositional view: Individual can determine if a mammal is or is not a dog, uses the term "dog" appropriately, and acts in an appropriate way when a dog is present.

CONCEPTUAL CHANGE OVER TIME

Although concepts are often thought of as being defined by strict criteria that do not change (referred to as *necessary and sufficient conditions*), there are numerous instances where this does not hold true. Furthermore, even for those instances that do seem to fit at present, the possibility and in fact the likelihood of change in the future needs to be instilled in students as a reminder to keep up to date with the latest knowledge. History is full of examples of situations in which there seemed good reason to believe that certainty had been achieved, only to have that certainty questioned over time. A student in astronomy who had a solid grasp of the concept of *Planet* probably was very comfortable with the classification of Pluto as a planet—until it was no longer classified that way. Ultimately, a newer concept of *Dwarf Planet* evolved, all the time building on a general idea of planet, but with the opportunity for change and refinement over time as new information about Pluto and other astronomical bodies was uncovered. The interplay of ideas led to a different understanding of the concepts of planet and dwart planet and, of course, the specific planet Pluto. Health care and nursing experience similar changes over time on an ongoing basis and, in fact, this change is essential to reflect emerging science.

Concepts in Nursing

HISTORICAL PERSPECTIVES: CONCEPTS FOR LEARNING AND CONCEPTS FOR THEORY

In nursing, concepts have been identified as important elements of knowledge for decades. Much of the work on concepts in nursing historically was focused on either how to make them clearer or the task of analyzing or synthesizing concepts as a way of developing the knowledge base. Catherine Norris (1982) was one of the first persons to focus on concepts in the context of the nursing knowledge base with her text *Concept Clarification in Nursing*. Since the late 1980s, the work of Walker and Avant (1988, 1995, 2005, 2011, 2019) has been a staple in graduate nursing courses oriented toward a discussion of theory in nursing. Along with Norris, Walker and Avant presented nurses with ideas about concept analysis and ushered in a particular focus on analysis that continues decades later. Chinn and Kramer (1991, 2011) also addressed concepts in their writings, particularly with regard to concept development, and Meleis (1991, 1997, 2007, 2012) has contributed a discussion of concepts and the role of concepts in the knowledge base of nursing.

Since the 1980s, the idea of concepts as "building blocks of theory" and an emphasis on concept analysis has been prevalent in the nursing literature. A myriad of publications have presented the results of analyses of concepts using diverse approaches and with varying levels of rigor. Although an extensive array of concepts has been addressed in this manner, and multiple analyses have been performed for many concepts, little effort has been expended to tie the analyses to substantive epistemic, scientific, or clinical problems in the discipline or to relate this content to teaching and learning. As a result, the literature abounds with articles on concepts and attempts to clarify concepts with minimal connection to how such approaches solve actual problems or enhance the knowledge base of the discipline (Rodgers, 1989, 2000). Because of the renewed emphasis on concepts in the context of the conceptual approach in nursing education, addressing the discussion of concepts in a substantive manner is imperative.

The prevailing thinking in nursing about concepts being primarily the "building blocks of theory" is found widely throughout nursing theory texts. Unfortunately, this emphasis leaves a lot of people thinking of concepts only in terms of theory, thus ignoring the critical role they play in learning overall. This perspective can also potentially give nursing faculty the impression that theory is needed for a curriculum to link the concepts together to have a sensible and useful knowledge base. Although the value of theory cannot be disputed, concepts themselves are powerful theoretical packages on their own and a theoretical umbrella for the curriculum is unnecessary. In the conceptual approach, the emphasis is placed on concepts at the level of individual learning rather than in regard to theory in general. That said, conceptual learning connects knowledge to action, and creates a logical linkage to a broader theory base to inform nursing practice.

A rich understanding regarding concepts along with agreement on a core of concepts that are essential to characterize nursing as a discipline and to provide a substantive basis for reasoned nursing action is needed. Concepts that are selected as the focus for nursing education send a message to students about the core areas of emphasis in the discipline. How those concepts are organized, the language used to communicate them, and the values that are expressed when a concept is shared with students have a considerable impact not only on the learning that takes place but also on the socialization of students to the profession of nursing.

WHY ARE CONCEPTS SO IMPORTANT FOR LEARNING?

The previous discussion about concept acquisition, behavior, and language reveals why concepts are important and are an appropriate focal point in education. Concepts are the objects of thought, and they are organizational elements for thinking. Because of common understandings of language, it is possible to communicate our ideas and concepts with others. It is important to recognize, however, that although different people might use the same word to describe a situation, it does not mean that they possess the same concept. In working with learners, it is important to determine appropriate means of assessment beyond the proper use of a word. It is also necessary to evaluate the thinking that underlies that term, in other words, the underlying concept. Nonetheless, without a connection between concepts and some form of expression (most commonly a formal language), communication is not possible. Similarly, without some connection between concepts and action, behavior and actions become random, isolated, and based on a case or situation, without the ability to apply knowledge across different situations. The critical point to remember is that the formation of concepts is essential to learning and to learned action; and the focus should be on concepts that are relevant, effective, and of practical use to the learner.

Transferable Learning

Because concepts are important organizational elements, they provide a way of clustering knowledge that enables someone with a strong grasp of a concept to draw on and apply what was learned in one situation to another situation; prior experiences and conceptual understanding helps that person interpret the new situation. Nurses cannot approach every encounter as a completely unique situation, nor can they manage each interaction as if it were an isolated case. It is necessary to have some way of grasping information cognitively and organizing it so it is available for application across varied encounters and new situations. Concepts serve that purpose. Furthermore, the application of concepts in a new situation allows the learner to refine their understanding of the concepts (Fig. 3.1).

Consider the concept of *Asepsis*. In a skills-oriented course, the nursing student will learn how to insert an indwelling urinary catheter and all of the appropriate steps in that process. The student also will learn about isolation technique, handwashing, and numerous other skills. If the student has a strong grasp of the concept of *Asepsis*, he or she can apply the cognitive content across a variety of situations. Without understanding the concept of *Asepsis*, the student is in a position of memorizing the steps of each procedure as if they were unrelated. A solid understanding of a concept enables the student to identify similarities across situations and transfer knowledge from one context to the next. The understanding

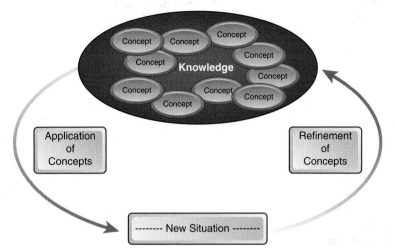

Fig. 3.1 Concepts are used to apply knowledge from one situation to another, resulting in concept refinement.

of *Asepsis* that accompanies having a good grasp of the concept enables the application of knowledge in a variety of situations.

Common Expression, Shared Understandings

The emphasis on knowledge and the ability to learn and carry information from one situation to the next are key aspects of a conceptual approach to teaching and learning. To enact such an approach, it is necessary to have a thorough understanding of what is meant by the term "concept." In other words, the educator, as well as the student, must have a meaningful concept of what a *concept* is. It is also important to understand how concepts are communicated and shared. Without some way to discuss concepts and share ideas, a conceptual approach to teaching and a concept-based curriculum would not be possible. Language and experience also need to be considered because they are important components of an understanding of concepts.

The implications of this approach are easy to see with regard to concepts that relate to physical objects. For example, nurses learn about thermometers as part of their education, and an actual physical object exists that can be held in the nurse's hand and is referred to using the term "thermometer." In this case, the word "thermometer" is the proper name of such an object. *Thermometer* can also represent a concept that is not any specific thermometer but is an idea the nurse possesses about any number of similar physical objects. If the nurse grasps the concept of *Thermometer*, in other words, recognizes the cluster of characteristics, abstracted from the physical objects and representative of all items that can be referred to as "thermometer," the nurse can understand the function and basic operation of any such device even though they do not all look and operate in the same way. Because such physical objects do exist, the teacher might evaluate the individual's concept by determining whether the learner can identify related objects successfully (i.e., thermometers), communicate about them, and differentiate thermometers from other devices.

Although the example concerning the concept of *Thermometer* is straightforward, most concepts featured in a concept-based curriculum in nursing pertain to nonphysical occurrences, such as the concept of *Professionalism*. The concept is formed on the basis of a cluster of characteristics or attributes, and although there is not a physical object that can be pointed to as "professionalism," there are experiences with examples of these concepts that can be provided through the educational process and by way of role modeling and observation. The nursing student can develop a grasp of the concept of *Professionalism* through these encounters and thus have a broader understanding rather than knowledge that is based on specific cases or situations. It does not serve the student well if he or she can only point to a particular person as being professional or not, or someone who acts in a professional manner. Instead, students need to understand what it is to be *Professional* and then be able to apply that across a variety of circumstances. This surely seems like a very abstract idea, but it represents the difference between understanding how to label something and treating words as names or in grasping the abstract learning that guides the use of words.

MISCONCEPTIONS AND CLARIFICATIONS

Misconception: Defining a concept is the same as defining how a word is used or stating the meaning of the word.

Clarification: The definition of the concept is based on the attributes that are clustered together to form the concept. Then a word or term is used to communicate the concept. The concept is the idea or the thinking that is expressed using the word. Meaning is the individual, personal interpretation that a person places on the concept. It is an important part of learning, but it is not the same as definition.

Developing Concepts for Nursing Education

When faculty commit to adopting a conceptual approach, the curriculum foundation is created by selecting relevant concepts to be used. Faculty also determine the focus of each concept in terms of definitions, use, and language. For each concept selected, several aspects need to be considered: How is the concept defined and presented to the students? In what settings do instances of the concept occur? What effect does context/setting/user have on the concept? What other concepts are similar, related, or easily confused with the concept of interest? How is that concept expressed or shared or discussed with others? What means are appropriate to assess a student's grasp of the concept? Other chapters in this text discuss various aspects of these challenges. In this section, the focus is on definitions, relationships among concepts, and language, because these components are critical to the formation of learning and evaluation strategies as a foundation for developing and implementing a sound curriculum for concept-based teaching.

DEFINING THE CONCEPTS

Nursing faculty are familiar with the common use of the term "definition." Dictionaries of all shapes and sizes are full of definitions that address the common purpose of using a word in a particular way to promote communication. In simple terms, a definition of a word may be referred to as the "meaning" of that word, similar to its reference or proper use in a sentence. Knowing the definition of a word enables a person to use that word effectively in a sentence and, if the person on the receiving end understands that definition, that individual can understand what the speaker or writer is trying to convey. When the number of homonyms in the English language is considered, the need for definitions of this type becomes clear (Box 3.2). Homonyms also point out the importance of making a distinction between concepts and the words that are used to express those concepts. The words may be the same, but in many cases, the concepts expressed by the word can be very different.

Because a concept is composed of a set of attributes, a conceptual definition incorporates a clear statement of those attributes. A definition can be considered adequate, or more appropriately "conceptually adequate," when it stipulates the components of the concept with sufficient clarity that the concept can be used effectively (Rodgers, 2000). Concepts in nursing generally have a core set of attributes that are stable over time, however, as mentioned previously, concepts can evolve over time as new evidence is gained (Fig. 3.2). For example, the concept of *Infection* can be defined by stating the attributes that are essential to identify, without a doubt, an instance of actual infection. This concept has been in existence for a long time and has a definition that is consistent and is applicable across a variety of contexts. As new evidence is gained about infection over time, changes are likely to be seen in terms of risk factors, protective mechanisms, and other aspects that influence the course and outcome of infection. A conceptually adequate definition of the concept of *Infection*, then, will provide the revised attributes that are appropriate to recognizing infection and understanding the contextual factors that lead to and follow its occurrence. The likelihood of future changes to concepts needs to be instilled in students as a reminder to keep up to date with the latest knowledge.

BOX 3.2 ■ Homonyms

A homonym is a word with the same spelling and pronunciation but with different definitions. A homonym does not usually express the same *concept*. Each use of the term must be associated with a different concept and conceptual definition for correct application. Consider all the following applications for the concept of *Bill*:

- Money; a dollar bill
- The part of a bird's jaw with a horny covering; a beak
- An itemized statement of fees or charges
- The visor portion of a cap
- A common first name
- A draft of proposed law presented for legislation

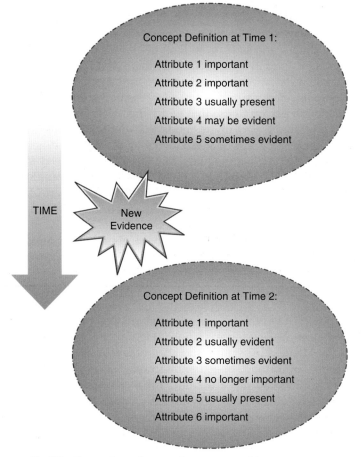

Fig. 3.2 Concepts evolve over time as new evidence emerges.

Essentialism and Probabilism

Another important aspect of concepts concerns how rigid and clear in definition a concept is required to be. When concepts are confused with words or specific objects, the tendency will be to think of the concept as having a very clear and rigid definition. Although all views of concepts focus on the attributes that compose the concept, the extent to which these are specific, clear, or unchanging does vary. In other words, concepts represent a continuum, with varying degrees of abstractness that affect how they are learned and applied. Philosophers refer to this as the *contrast of essentialism and probabilism.*

An essentialist position argues definitions are very rigid and clear. Essentialism, with regard to concepts, means that the attributes are both necessary and sufficient to define the concept. If any aspect is missing, the situation is not an example of that concept. By contrast, a probabilistic view focuses on a core of attributes that are *generally* required, but there is a bit of fuzziness that allows for some judgment as well as acknowledgment that concepts evolve over time as new evidence emerges (see Fig. 3.2).

Concepts and Taxonomies

One place where a more rigid form of definition is helpful is in the area of taxonomies. A taxonomy is a classification system. The more rigid end of that continuum is anchored by concepts that have very specific criteria that are either present, or not, to be an example of the concept. Because the definitions are stipulated, with very precise criteria, a different type of learning may be facilitated, and faculty might expect more stringent application of criteria. Even in the case of taxonomies, which involve strictly prescribed definitions, there can be challenges in the attempt to create categories that are mutually exclusive and without overlap. In some fields this task is easier to achieve, such as in the classification of biologic organisms (e.g., flowers or insects). In situations involving humans, however, criteria often are presented in the form of a list in which only some of the items on the list must be present for the label to be applicable, thus indicating that there is no single core of characteristics that is captured by the concept.

As an example, some disease categories fall into taxonomies and have strict criteria that determine whether the specific medical diagnosis applies. A nurse may have a clear concept of *Dementia*, but this may not be exactly the same as a diagnosis of dementia. This just presents another example of how concepts, words, taxonomies all can vary. With conceptual learning, the emphasis on the concept provides the critical foundation on which it is possible to build word use, diagnoses, and other related ideas. A solid understanding of the concept provides an organizing structure to understand taxonomies, diagnoses, and variations of the condition being addressed. Diagnostic categories change on the basis of new knowledge and changes in social norms, and thus these taxonomies must be reconstructed periodically.

THE NEED FOR CONCEPTUAL CLARITY

A critical aspect of the conceptual approach is determining what concepts are essential for the curriculum and how those concepts will be presented—in other words, what will constitute a "conceptually adequate" approach for the purposes of the educational setting. Providing students with a list of essential attributes, thus invoking the idea of "necessary and sufficient conditions" or an unchanging set of attributes, gives students the impression that concepts are static, with distinguishable boundaries, and with consistency regardless of context or situation. This approach promotes memorization rather than application because students undoubtedly will be focused on learning the essential attributes so those can be recited at a later time (e.g., on multiple choice tests).

What is needed for teaching purposes is for students to identify and communicate core features (attributes) of a concept while allowing for other considerations such as application, variation across contexts, and conceptual change. Although students may strive for some sort of absolute answer to all information presented, part of their learning is understanding and appreciating that concepts must be amenable to variation across individuals, cultures, contexts, and the variation required by new discoveries.

CONCEPT ANALYSIS AND CLARIFICATION

The process of identifying the core components of a concept is referred to as concept clarification, which most commonly is accomplished through a concept analysis. Concept analysis is the process of breaking a concept down to identify the attributes that constitute its definition. It also involves identifying other aspects of the concept, particularly contextual factors, that are important in being able to use the concept effectively. Because concepts have an important "use," it is possible to look at how it is used in the context of healthcare to determine what makes up the concept.

Concept analysis is well established in the literature of nursing, and several different methodologies exist for this purpose. Box 3.3 contains a list of some of the methodologies that have been used in nursing studies. Exploring concepts for purposes of concept-based teaching may not be formal research, but it still calls for rigorous and sound inquiry. Similarly, the process and the presentation of the concept to students needs to be consistent throughout the curriculum.

In selecting the approach to clarify a concept for purposes of concept-based teaching, the instructor also should consider the nature of the concept to be analyzed. Some concepts are suited to more specificity, such as those that are represented by diagnostic criteria or taxonomies. It also may be possible to identify physical or tangible objects that serve as examples of such concepts, which can make clarification and description easier to accomplish, keeping in mind actual objects that represent the concept. Morse et al. (1996) referred to some concepts as being "mature" in reference to the length of their existence and presumed state of development. It is often assumed that more mature concepts are capable of greater precision because of their longevity. However, a lengthy period of use predisposes a concept to more variation and change over time. For the purposes of concept-based teaching, the most likely sources of data for examining the use of the concept are the professional literature, such as journal publications and textbooks. Many of the concepts of interest to faculty for inclusion in the curricula may have completed analyses available in the nursing or health sciences literature.

BOX 3.3 ■ Approaches to Concept Analysis Used in Nursing

- Morse (1995)—Principle-Based Concept Analysis
- Norris (1982)—Concept Clarification
- Walker and Avant (1983, 2011)—Concept Analysis
- Rodgers (1989, 2000)—Evolutionary Cycle of Concept Development
- Schwartz-Barcott and Kim (1986)—Hybrid Model of Concept Development

USING THE EVOLUTIONARY VIEW FOR CONCEPT ANALYSIS

The Evolutionary View is associated with a formal process of concept analysis that can be used in a thorough attempt at concept clarification for the purposes of teaching. This approach looks similar to the one advocated by the popular writings of Walker and Avant (2011). In fact, all approaches to concept analysis have a great deal in common regarding the specific activities that are conducted as part of the analysis. There are, however, what may seem subtle but actually are quite profound differences.

For purposes of developing clear concepts for the conceptual approach, the Evolutionary View process can be very effective. Note that it also can be used in teaching, taking students through the process of the analysis to ensure that all of the components of the concept are presented clearly through the learning experience. For a thorough discussion of this approach, please see the description provided elsewhere (Rodgers, 2000). A simplified four-step version, intended for ease of use by instructors and faculty, is provided below. It is important to point out that the following sections could give the impression that the process occurs in sequential fashion. However, the process of concept clarification is not a linear process at all! Each activity discussed can be affected by all the others; for example, determining what terminology will work best for a literature review will be affected by the literature that is uncovered during the review. This terminology may again need to be changed as literature is reviewed. It is important to see the flow of activities as an iterative process, with each activity influenced by the others.

MISCONCEPTIONS AND CLARIFICATIONS

Misconception: The various approaches to concept analysis found in the literature are essentially the same.

Clarification: The various approaches to concept analysis appear similar in many ways, but the differences actually are quite profound.

Identify the Concept of Interest

First, it is essential to identify the concept of interest. The emphasis needs to be on the idea that is communicated, not the specific word that is used to discuss it. Words are expressions of ideas, not the ideas themselves. It is important to be clear about what the concept of interest is and then explore what term is best used to express that concept. The selection of the term will guide the clarification process, along with any teaching and learning interactions with students. It is possible that two terms express similar ideas, and it may be appropriate to explore both to determine which term is most appropriate and has the broadest support. As an example, the terms "grief" and "bereavement" both have relevance in the exploration of the same concept, although a thorough review of the literature does reveal some differences (Cowles and Rodgers, 2000). In selecting the concepts to be included in the curriculum, and in discriminating among closely related concepts, students are being socialized into the discipline and profession of nursing (Toulmin, 1972). The concepts that are chosen as the focus for the curriculum will shape the development of students as professional nurses.

Determine the Relevant Context

The process of concept clarification and development requires attention to the context – meaning how the concept is used or appears in practice. As an example, in the context of health care, *coping* refers to behavioral and cognitive means of adjusting to various situations. *Coping,* as a concept, involves not only a positive outcome, as in, "She is coping well with her new challenges," but the process of making responses to changing stimuli. *Coping* often is discussed in health care in the context of other concepts such as *Stress, Adaptation,* and *Resilience* (Buchanan, 2021). The term "coping" also can be found in regard to woodworking, such as "coping saw" (Walker and Avant, 2011). In some respects, this concept is similar, because the saw makes precise and fine adjustments to produce intricate patterns in the material being cut. The saw makes it possible for wood, for example, to respond to its surroundings to make a precise fit. Some scholars would argue that all varied uses of the same concept should be included in the analysis. However, this approach would be misleading on a number of levels because these uses and ideas of coping clearly miss the intricacies and important aspects of coping as a psychological and cognitive process (Buchanan, 2021; Rodgers, 2000). Furthermore, this approach is a solid example of confusing terminology, or the use of a word, with the use of a concept. Keeping the focus on the concept of *Coping* in the context of nursing practice will help students focus and ensure a clear emphasis on the concept of interest rather than on the terminology. Settings and application also may include considerations about age, culture, and care context, to the extent that those considerations are relevant. These applications are just a few in a long list of possible applications that exist for many concepts of interest in nursing.

Collect Data to Clarify the Concept

Data collection proceeds once some of the critical decisions about the concept have been made. The data collection process may lead the faculty to look at other terminology, sources, or contexts. Consequently, even though data collection is a major focus of the concept analysis and development processes, it is not an isolated endeavor that is pursued without regard for the other parts of the process. Data collection is focused on collecting sufficient information to determine the major components of the concept. These components include the attributes of the concept—in other words, its key components—along with discussion of the context in which the concept is used. Context can include social and cultural considerations in addition to elements that reflect a time sequence. Situations or events that occur before an instance of the concept and those that occur after are typically discussed as "antecedents" and "consequences," respectively. Antecedents and consequences help to put the concept in an application setting so that students can understand not just the concept but when they might see examples of it and what creates a situation in which the concept is applicable, along with possible outcomes. Data that help answer these questions are derived from the literature and then are analyzed to develop clear indicators of the effective use of the concept. Proceeding in this manner reveals the "state of the science" regarding the concept for application in nursing (Rodgers, 2000).

Identify Exemplars

A fourth step is the identification of concept exemplars, which will help students grasp the application of the concept in the appropriate context. The term "exemplar" is used purposefully in the Evolutionary Method to reflect the fact that these examples ideally can be found in "real life" and are not models or paradigmatic cases that are constructed by the person doing the analysis (Fehr, 1988; Rodgers, 2000). Multiple exemplars are used to show the nuances of the concept in different applications and contexts and to help students accept how boundaries can be fuzzy and unclear as opposed to always distinct and rigid.

Important to note, an exemplar is not the same as a "model case." A model case, according to Wilson (1963), is a case "which we are absolutely sure is an instance of the concept in that it contains all of the conditions that are necessary and sufficient to comprise an example of the concept" (p. 28). Walker and Avant (2011) include these and other types of cases in their approach to analysis. There is a significant problem with "model" cases, however, in that they may give the impression of greater clarity and certainty than is appropriate.

A FINAL NOTE ABOUT CONDUCTING CONCEPT ANALYSIS FOR THE CONCEPTUAL APPROACH

The preceding section outlined four steps to conduct a concept analysis for concepts in a concept-based curriculum. However, it is not necessary to pursue this in-depth process of concept clarification for every concept addressed in the curriculum. It would be prohibitive to do a formal analysis, using a rigorous sample drawn from the literature, for every concept that will be discussed. Fortunately, references and textbooks exist that present some of the work that has been done along these lines. In addition, a literature search will uncover an extensive number of articles presenting the results of analyses although, as with all research, the quality of the studies varies. For concepts that are particularly confusing or vague or the focal point of disagreement among the faculty, a formal analysis may be of benefit. Even if a formal analysis is not completed, however, the faculty need to be comfortable presenting the key elements of the concept and can structure the presentation according to the aspects of the concept that are essential for understanding.

BRINGING THE CONCEPT PRESENTATION TO LIFE

The results of concept analysis, when reported in the literature, may seem very tedious or cumbersome to read. There typically is a listing of each of the major components with varying amounts of discussion about each component. For purposes of inquiry, where it is necessary to be clear about the status of each component of the concept to identify directions for future development, this information may be useful. For education, however, it is more important that the concept be presented in a way that comes alive for students. The necessary degree of conceptual clarity must be present, but the analysis and presentation will be more effective if the components are woven together in a manner that helps students grasp the appearance and use of the concept in real-life situations.

The intent of concept clarification activities in a concept-based curriculum is to help the students grasp the concept and be able to use it effectively. This includes giving students sufficient information to (1) recognize the occurrence of the concept and be clear and appropriate in its application; (2) value the contextual elements; (3) recognize and use associated terminology; (4) explore distinctions among similar concepts; and (5) appreciate the nuances and subtleties of the concept and its areas of imperfection. There is no limit to how a concept can be presented to help students grasp these components. Whatever the focus of discussion, however, there must be a "conceptually adequate" definition that demonstrates the prevailing attributes of the concept and its scope of application.

Case studies can be an important strategy to help students grasp the concept, but it is important not to fall into the trap of "model cases." Model cases, as noted previously, can place inappropriate boundaries on a concept and cause the individual learning the concept to assume too narrow a scope of application. The learner may reach the conclusion that, if such an example is a model, then *all* instances of the concept will appear to be similar. Even relatively clear-cut concepts, such as *Mobility*, have numerous variations related to arthritis, postoperative ambulation, amputation, and many more instances, in addition to the positive aspects such as athleticism. Focusing on a model case of *Mobility*, perhaps in the case of a distance runner who clearly is very "mobile," will present an unnecessary and unrealistic example that does not show the range of use of the concept and its relevance in numerous instances in nursing.

Summary

The conceptual approach matches an important part of the natural process of learning, provides a foundation and skills for life-long development, creates receptivity and openness to change consistent with a dynamic knowledge base, and emphasizes the knowledge that underlies practice rather than merely the jobs or roles in which nurses perform. For such an approach to be successful, however, it is essential that the faculty have an understanding of the nature of concepts and how they function in the process of learning and be consistent in their philosophical viewpoint about concepts. Faculty also need to recognize the importance of conceptual change in the discipline and connect that to evidence-based practice. Doing so will provide the students not only with a foundation of concepts essential for nursing practice but an appreciation for adapting to new developments in the discipline as they arise.

Methods of concept development, particularly concept analysis and clarification, are essential in a concept-based curriculum. Following a documented approach to clarification can help ensure that the appropriate components of a concept are understood well, presented clearly, and described in relevant contexts similar to how students are expected to use the concepts. Essential components of a concept, which are sufficient to provide a high degree of clarity, can be articulated within a concept development framework. This can provide a structure for presentation and discussion, as well as for making sure that all critical aspects are addressed. It is important, however, that the approach to analysis and clarification be one that promotes critical thinking, relevant application, and a strong grasp of the concept as demonstrated by the students' ability to use the concept effectively (Rodgers, 2000).

References

Ambrose SA, Bridges MW, DiPietro M, et al. *How Learning Works. 7 Research-Based Principles for Smart Teaching.* San Francisco, CA: Jossey-Bass; 2010.

Buchanan L. Stress and coping. In: Giddens JF, ed. *Concepts for Nursing Practice.* 3rd ed. St. Louis, MO: Mosby; 2021:300–316. 291.

Chinn PL, Kramer MK. *Integrated Theory and Knowledge Development in Nursing.* 8th ed. St. Louis, MO: Elsevier; 2011.

Chinn PL, Kramer MK. *Theory and Nursing: A Systematic Approach.* 3rd ed. St. Louis, MO: Mosby; 1991.

Cowles KV, Rodgers BL. The concept of grief: an evolutionary perspective. In: Rodgers BL, Knafl KA, eds. *Concept Development in Nursing: Foundations Techniques, and Applications.* Philadelphia, PA: Saunders; 2000:103–117.

Erickson L, Lanning LA, French R. *Concept-Based Curriculum and Instruction for the Thinking Classroom.* Thousand Oaks, CA: Corwin Press; 2017.

Fehr B. Prototype analysis of the concepts of love and commitment. *J Pers Soc Psycho.* 1988;55:557–579.

Lizardo O. Re-conceptualizing abstract conceptualization in social theory: the case of the "structure" concept. *J Theory Soc Behav.* 2013;43(2):155–180.

Mahon BZ, Caramazza A. Concepts and categories: a cognitive neuropsychological perspective. *Ann Rev Psychol.* 2009;60:27–51.

Meleis AI. *Theoretical Nursing.* 2nd ed. Philadelphia, PA: J. B. Lippincott; 1991.

Meleis AI. *Theoretical Nursing.* 3rd ed. Philadelphia, PA: J. B. Lippincott; 1997.

Meleis AI. *Theoretical Nursing.* 4th ed. Philadelphia, PA: Lippincott Williams & Wilkins; 2007.

Meleis AI. *Theoretical Nursing.* 5th ed. Philadelphia, PA: Lippincott Williams & Wilkins; 2012.

Morse JM. Exploring the theoretical basis of nursing knowledge using advanced techniques of concept analysis. *Adv Nurs Sci.* 1995;17:31–46.

Morse JM, Mitcham C, Hupcey JE, et al. Criteria for concept evaluation. *J Adv Nurs.* 1996;24:385–390.

Norris CM. *Concept Clarification in Nursing.* Rockville, MD: Aspen; 1982.

Renkl A. Instruction based on examples. In: Mayer RE, Alexander PA, eds. *Handbook of Research on Learning and Instruction.* New York: Routledge; 2017.

Rodgers BL. Concepts, analysis, and the development of nursing knowledge: the evolutionary cycle. *J Adv Nurs.* 1989;14:330–335.

Rodgers BL. Philosophical foundations of concept development. In: Rodgers BL, Knafl KA, eds. *Concept Development in Nursing: Foundations, Techniques, and Applications.* Philadelphia, PA: W. B. Saunders; 2000:7–37.

Schwartz-Barcott D, Kim HS. A hybrid model for concept development. In: Chinn P, ed. *Nursing Research Methodology: Issues and Implementation.* Rockville, MD: Aspen; 1986:91–101.

Sundbo DIC. Local food: the social construction of a concept, Section B, soil and plant science. *Acta Agric Scand B.* 2013;63(suppl 1):66–77.

Timpson WM, Bendel-Simso P. *Concepts and Choices for Teaching: Meeting the Challenges in Higher Education.* Madison, WI: Magna Publications; 1996.

Toulmin S. *Human Understanding.* Princeton, NJ: Princeton University; 1972.

Walker LO, Avant KC. *Strategies for Theory Construction in Nursing.* Norwalk, CT: Appleton-Century-Crofts; 1983.

Walker LO, Avant KC. *Strategies for Theory Construction in Nursing.* 2nd ed. Norwalk, CT: Appleton & Lange; 1988.

Walker LO, Avant KC. *Strategies for Theory Construction in Nursing.* 3rd ed. Norwalk, CT: Appleton & Lange; 1995.

Walker LO, Avant KC. *Strategies for Theory Construction in Nursing.* 4th ed. Upper Saddle River, NJ: Pearson Education; 2005.

Walker LO, Avant KC. *Strategies for Theory Construction in Nursing.* 5th ed. Upper Saddle River, NJ: Pearson Education; 2011.

Walker LO, Avant KC. *Strategies for Theory Construction in Nursing.* 5th ed. Upper Saddle River, NJ: Pearson Education; 2019.

Wilson J. *Thinking With Concepts.* London, UK: Cambridge University Press; 1963.

CHAPTER 4

Developing a Concept-Based Curriculum

One of the key elements for the successful adoption of the conceptual approach is the development of a concept-based curriculum. The term *curriculum* refers to the arrangement of content within courses that form an academic program. In a concept-based curriculum, concepts provide the foundation for the organizational structure of the curriculum. Curriculum development follows a standard, predictable process, regardless of the discipline, the type of learning program, or the level of the learner. A curriculum should align with the overarching goals of the academic institution and nursing school and should support learner attainment of identified program learning outcomes.

Collectively, program faculty are responsible for the development, implementation, and evaluation of a curriculum that is effective and efficient; furthermore, faculty must ensure that the curriculum meets current professional nursing standards, policies, and regulatory requirements. Faculty are also well-served to maintain an awareness of trends and changes in healthcare, higher education, and the general society to ensure that the curriculum is contemporary and relevant. The rapid changes in health care alone affect the need for regular curriculum revision to maintain currency. Curriculum work is a complex, ongoing process that is time consuming and requires attention to many details. Most faculty have not had formal instruction in curriculum design and evaluation which can create challenges, unless a seasoned educator can lead the work (Hopkins and Kroning, 2021). Faculty development in curriculum development and revision is an area of opportunity for most nursing schools. Several books dedicated solely to the art of curriculum development, revision, and evaluation are helpful references for faculty; however, such detail is beyond the scope of this chapter. This chapter provides a general overview of curriculum development and revision and incorporates unique elements associated with a conceptual approach.

Overview: Curriculum Development and Revision

The purpose of a curriculum is to provide an organizational structure to the content within an academic program so that learners can successfully achieve predetermined learning outcomes. A curriculum includes a group of elements to provide that structure, including program goals and outcomes, curriculum framework, courses, and an evaluation process.

The terms *"curriculum development"* and *"curriculum revision"* are often used interchangeably but have different meanings. Curriculum development typically refers to the process of creating a new curriculum. A new curriculum is needed when preparing for a new academic program or when a decision is made to retire an existing curriculum for a program and create a new one, starting with a "clean slate." This is typically needed when adopting a new curriculum framework and model. The adoption of a new concept-based curriculum generally involves the development of a new curriculum. Curriculum revision refers to the process of updating and revising an existing curriculum without changing the framework or model. Curriculum revision can range from major (eliminating courses, adopting new courses, changing credit hours, major changes to program outcomes, etc.) to minor (revisions to courses, prerequisites, minor edits to program outcomes).

Curriculum work is not a one-time event; rather it represents a continuous quality improvement philosophy. As shown in Fig. 4.1, the curriculum life cycle begins with the decision to develop a new curriculum or revise an existing curriculum based on evaluation data and/or external contextual factors. After a curriculum is developed or revised, a series of approvals are required before it can be implemented. The type of approval needed and specific approval process will vary from institution to institution, depending on if the curriculum proposal represents a new program, a significant or major curriculum revision, or minor revisions to an existing curriculum. At a minimum, the curriculum approval process requires faculty approval within the school as a function of shared governance

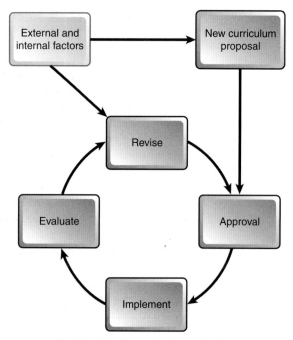

Fig. 4.1   The life cycle of a curriculum.

outlined in faculty bylaws. A new curriculum proposal or a curriculum proposal reflecting major revisions will need institutional approval and may also need approval by the state and/or by other regulatory agencies.

Implementation of the new or revised curriculum occurs only after gaining formal approval (see Fig. 4.1). A recruitment plan is developed to ensure adequate student enrollment, and the nursing school offers the new and/or revised courses according to the program of study for the new curriculum. There may also be a need for a "teach out" plan if students admitted under a previous curriculum are still enrolled. Evaluation of student learning occurs as part of course delivery in the curriculum.

The final step in the curriculum lifecycle includes program evaluation. Data are regularly collected as part of a program evaluation plan and are analyzed by the faculty. Program evaluation reports are reviewed and discussed, which in turn provides evidence for future curriculum revisions as they are needed.

The general curriculum development and revision process presented here applies to any type of curriculum (including a concept-based curriculum) in any academic program in any discipline. A deeper dive into the multiple steps associated with curriculum development are presented in the following sections.

Foundational Elements

INTERNAL AND EXTERNAL CONTEXT FOR CURRICULUM CHANGE

It is often said that faculty "own" the curriculum, meaning that faculty are accountable for continually developing, implementing, evaluating, and revising the curriculum. Several internal and external factors and issues play a significant role in the curriculum; thus, nurse educators must remain vigilant to such issues and factors.

Internal factors include the expertise of the faculty in curriculum development, program outcomes, other curricula offered by a nursing school or department, institutional policies, institutional culture, student characteristics, physical resources, and human resources (e.g., the number of faculty, staff, and students enrolled). Specific to the conceptual approach, one of the most important internal contexts to consider is faculty expertise. Expertise is needed for appropriate decision-making and to clearly articulate the conceptual approach to administrators, other faculty, students, and external stakeholders.

External factors include professional practice standards, accreditation standards, regulatory bodies, and clinical agencies; these external drivers of change may also have policy implications. Several external factors that have recently influenced curriculum change in nursing include seminal position statements and reports such as *The Future of Nursing 2020–2030: Charting a Path to Achieve Health Equity* (National Academies of Sciences, Engineering, and Medicine [NASEM], 2021), *AACN's Vision for Academic Nursing* (American Association of Colleges of Nursing [AACN], 2019); *The Essentials: Core Competencies for Professional Nursing Education* (AACN, 2021); *Educating Nurses: A Radical Call for Transformation* (Benner et al., 2010); *Registered Nurses: Partners in Transforming*

Primary Care (Josiah Macy Foundation, 2016); and *Achieving Competency-Based Time-Variable Health Professions Education* (Lucey, 2018). Additionally, the rapid of expansion of educational technologies, especially for online learning and simulation (Haydon et al., 2014; INACSL Standards Committee, 2016), has implications for curriculum development. Characteristics of the community served (such as population demographics and culture), socioeconomic factors, health care access, and employer demand represent other important external factors that are considered when designing or revising a curriculum.

External factors especially important to consider when adopting a conceptual approach are the perspectives of the employers and nurses within the community. It is essential that this group of stakeholders understand why the curriculum is changing and how it is envisioned; eliciting their support and input is critical. Most employers welcome a change in the educational system, especially if it means that nursing graduates will have higher-level thinking and problem-solving skills. Communicating the competencies of graduates is important for prospective employers. Nurses who interface directly or indirectly with students, must have an understanding of the changes that will occur, especially with regard to clinical education. Most nurses welcome a change in the educational system if it means that clinical education is less burdensome to the practice areas and if their input is solicited.

MISSION, VISION, AND VALUES

As a starting point for curriculum development, faculty should intentionally review and discuss the institutional mission and vision statements of the parent institution, as well as those stated by the nursing school or department. A mission statement explains organizational purpose or meaning; better stated, the mission statement describes why an entity exists. A vision is a statement of what an entity wants to be or what it wishes to accomplish. Thus, the mission and vision statements serve as a compass for the parent institution, as well as the nursing school or department. Consistency and clear linkages between the nursing school mission and vision and the institutional mission and vision statements are required (Fig. 4.2). It is possible that changes to the mission and vision are proposed as a result of the review, although this is not the primary intent. The primary benefit of such a discussion is the opportunity for faculty to gain a shared understanding and level-setting regarding the context for the curriculum work. In addition, a school's statement of values or beliefs provides consistency and integrity to all curriculum elements (Csokasy, 2002). These values and beliefs, held collectively by the faculty, guide actions and decision-making related to curriculum development and academic delivery.

PROGRAM GOALS AND PROGRAM LEARNING OUTCOMES

After the mission, vision, and values have been reviewed and discussed, members of the curriculum committee should develop or revise the program goals and the learning outcomes. Nursing schools that offer more than one academic

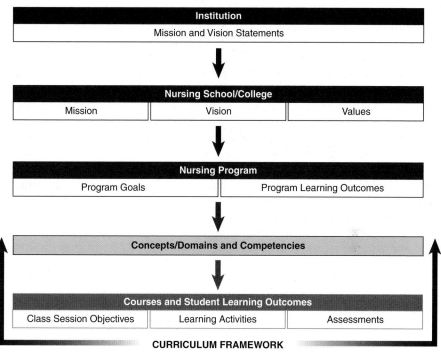

Fig. 4.2 Elements associated with a curriculum.

program (i.e., baccalaureate, master's, practice doctorate, and PhD) have program goals and program learning outcomes for each program. Program goals are broad-based statements that describe the overarching purpose of a program—why that program exists. For example, *"Prepare students for a rewarding career in professional nursing practice"* could serve as an overarching goal for a baccalaureate prelicensure nursing program.

Program learning outcomes (also referred to as end-of-program outcomes) serve as the expected characteristics of graduates after completing an academic program (Whittmann-Price and Fasolka, 2010). The term "outcome" refers to the end result of a process; thus, a program learning outcome is a specific statement that describes what a student will be able to do in a measurable way by the time he or she completes the program. Program learning outcomes are influenced by external forces (such as seminal reports and changes in educational or accreditation standards mentioned in the previous section). As a matter of sequence, faculty should consider identifying the program goals and program learning outcomes after reviewing and discussing the mission, vision, and values—and before developing the organizational framework.

Faculty often wonder if the process for developing program learning outcomes is different when developing a concept-based curriculum. Distinctions in curriculum primarily occur with curriculum design; thus, the same program learning outcomes could support a variety of curricular designs. For example, a common program learning outcome of an undergraduate curriculum may read something like this:

> *Collaborate as a member of an interdisciplinary team to improve the quality of health care.*

Such an outcome could be the desired expectation of any nursing graduate from any nursing program, regardless of the type of curricular design of the nursing program. However, the curricular design is the vehicle faculty choose to ensure that students can achieve this learning outcome. Thus, the *process* for developing program learning outcomes for a concept-based curriculum is the same as what would be done for any other curricular design, although the design should be taken into account to ensure that the structure fits the identified learning outcomes.

MISCONCEPTIONS AND CLARIFICATIONS

Misconception: Program learning outcomes are written completely differently when developing a concept-based curriculum—focusing only on concepts.	*Clarification:* Program learning outcomes reflect what a student can do as a result of the program and are written similar to program learning outcomes of traditional curricular design. Curricular concepts should link to program learning outcomes.

Curriculum Framework and Design

The organizational framework of a curriculum is essentially the blueprint or design that provides structure and clarifies the scope of content and how the curricular elements interface with the curriculum approach. Developing the organizational framework includes identifying and defining the structural elements to gain a shared understanding of what these elements mean and how the elements are constructed so that program learning outcomes are achievable. In addition, developing a clear plan about how the curriculum elements link together is critical. A visual model of the curricular framework shows the association among the elements within a curriculum and can be helpful to faculty and students to gain a better understanding of the curriculum. However, Boland advises a "less-is-more" principle related to the development of curricular models, warning that too complex of a model leads faculty to "spend more time trying to interpret and understand the framework than they do actually implementing and evaluating it" (Boland, 2012, p. 144).

One of the truly unique hallmarks of developing a concept-based curriculum is the curricular framework and design. The key elements of a concept-based curriculum framework include concepts (organized within concept categories) and the related competencies. The general process for developing the curricular design for a conceptual approach involves selecting and defining the concepts and concept categories, developing competencies (used as outcome measures for each concept), and then determining exemplars, course design, and program evaluation. The structural elements of the curriculum (concepts and competencies)

TABLE 4.1 ■ Linkages between Program Learning Outcomes, Concepts, Competencies, and Course Learning Outcomes in a Concept-Based Curriculum

Curricular Element	Example
Program learning outcome	Collaborate as a member of an interdisciplinary team to improve the quality of health care.
Curriculum concepts	• Collaboration • Quality and Safety
Competencies	• Assesses own understanding of collaboration to determine strengths and weaknesses as an effective member of a health care team. • Appraises the effectiveness and appropriateness of collaboration among members of the health care team in patient care delivery. • Incorporates the concepts of quality, safety, and collaboration into clinical experiences as a member of health care teams. • Effectively participates as a member of an interprofessional team to deliver safe and quality care.
Course learning outcomes	**NURS 317**: Describe the concepts of Health Care Quality, Safety, and Collaboration and their influences on healthcare delivery. **NURS 441**: Analyze the concepts of Health Care Quality, Safety, and Collaboration as foundational elements to effective healthcare delivery.

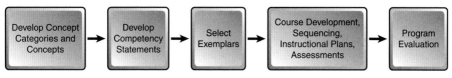

Fig. 4.3 Steps for concept-based curriculum design.

link to the program learning outcomes (Table 4.1) and drive course development, instruction, and assessments (representing a "backward design" approach). Fig. 4.3 shows these general steps and are discussed in further detail in the following sections.

CONCEPT CATEGORIES

Once the decision to adopt a concept-based curriculum is made, there is a tendency for faculty to immediately begin identifying and negotiating concepts to be included. However, a step that ideally precedes this process is the identification and development of concept categories. Concept categories provide structure to the curriculum through the organization of concepts and provide greater clarity about what the concepts represent. Development of the concept category involves establishing criteria or parameters regarding how concepts for each category are selected, identified, and applied. Parameters establish the "rules" or "criteria" involved in determining whether a concept fits within a category and also provide some guidelines regarding how it is framed and eventually taught. For example, concept categories might be related to patient populations, areas of health care practice, or even philosophical perspectives about health. Although the identification of concept categories ideally precedes selecting concepts using the deductive approach described, it is possible to select concepts first and then organize concepts to determine the broader concept categories—representing an inductive approach.

If a large number of concepts fit within a broad category, subcategories (or macroconcepts) are useful for further organization. As discussed in Chapter 1, a macroconcept represents a very broad concept and, in fact, usually represents multiple concepts (see Fig. 1.1). Concepts organized within a macroconcept are closely interrelated. The number and type of concept categories used within a curriculum can vary considerably and is one of the ways a curriculum from one school can distinguish itself from another. Three common concept categories are presented and described as examples in the following sections.

Health and Illness Concepts

Health and illness concepts represent a patient's health status in relation to three general goals of health care: the promotion of health, the prevention of disease, and the treatment of illness. These goals are interrelated and often thought of as a functional process. An established categorical description used to determine whether a concept fits in the category might be something as simple as *"A physiological or psychosocial health response."* Concepts such as *Gas Exchange*, *Infection*, *Mobility*, *Immunity*, *Cognition*, and *Mood* clearly fit, whereas concepts such as *Delegation*, *Policy*, and *Ethics* clearly do not. Health and illness concepts are considered from three contexts: *health continuum, life span continuum*, and *environment of care*. These contexts serve as guiding principles related to how the concepts are selected, presented, and applied (Fig. 4.4).

For example, the concept of *Immunity* represents conditions across the health-illness continuum (health promotion, acute illness, and chronic conditions) and across the life span continuum (infants, children, adolescents, adults, and older adults), and care delivery occurs across multiple environments (within hospital units and clinics, and from a community health perspective, public health perspective, and global perspective). Parameters such as these help with the selection process and provide clarity for use within the curriculum.

Because the health and illness concepts category is very large, macroconcepts help to further organize concepts; for example, a curriculum committee may wish to use a macroconcept such as Homeostasis and Regulation as a category for *Perfusion, Gas Exchange*, and *Hormonal Regulation*. Likewise, the concepts *Infection, Immunity, Mobility*, and *Tissue Integrity* logically fit under the macroconcept Protection and Movement (Table 4.2).

Professional Nursing Concepts

Concepts that represent the critical attributes and collectively describe professional nursing practice are called Professional Nursing concepts. These concepts are associated with professional comportment—or in other words, these

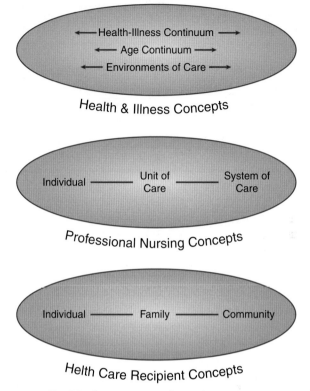

Fig. 4.4 Concept categories and parameters.

concepts link with the identity of nursing as a health care profession. Many of these concepts actually link more broadly to desired behaviors of all health care providers. Concepts such as *Professional Identity, Resilience, Cultural Humility, Health Policy,* and *Collaboration* all clearly fit in a category such as this.

Established parameters for the Professional Nursing Concept Category can be presented from the context of the *individual nurse,* the *unit of care,* and from a *system perspective* (see Fig. 4.4). For example, a concept such as *Health Policy* could be presented from the context of how policies affect a nurse in direct care (such as a uniform policy or a policy regarding central line care), how policies affect an organization (such as admission policies and reimbursement policies), and how policies affect the health care system. This concept could also be presented by taking one specific policy, such as the Health Insurance Portability and Accountability Act, and framing it from the context of the individual nurse, the organization, and the health care system.

Like the Health and Illness concepts, Professional Nursing concepts can be further organized with macroconcepts. For example, *Health Care Organizations, Health Care Economics, Health Policy,* and *Health Care Law* could be grouped under the macroconcept *Health Care Infrastructure.* Likewise, the concepts *Patient-Centered Care, Ethics, Diversity, Equity,* and *Inclusion* could logically fit under the macroconcept *Holistic Care* (Table 4.3).

TABLE 4.2 ■ **Example of Health and Illness Concept Category With Associated Macroconcepts and Concepts**

Concept Category	Macro-Concept	Examples of Concepts
Health and Illness Concepts	Homeostasis and Regulation	Perfusion, Gas Exchange, Hormonal Regulation, Thermoregulation, Acid-Base Balance
	Protection and Movement	Immunity, Inflammation, Tissue Integrity Mobility, Fatigue
	Mood, Cognition, Behavior	Stress and Coping, Anxiety, Cognition, Substance Misuse, Interpersonal Violence

Health Care Recipient Concepts

The healthcare delivery system has made major strides, particularly during the past two decades, to move from a disease-centered perspective (in which the health care providers control all aspects of care) to a patient-centered model whereby recipients of care are not only informed of care options but are partners in the care decisions. Delivery of patient-centered care requires recognizing that health care recipients are very diverse, and thus health care decisions must take into account the unique needs and preferences of the patient (Institute of Medicine [IOM], 2001; National Academies of Sciences, Engineering, and Medicine [NASEM], 2021; Ortiz, 2018).

As a concept category, health care recipient concepts represent the unique and distinct attributes of all health care recipients. It is essential for nurses to understand these fundamental concepts for the successful delivery of patient-centered care. For organizational purposes, it may be useful to use the macroconcepts *Personal Preferences* and *Attributes and Resources* to further categorize concepts in this category (Table 4.4).

TABLE 4.3 ■ **Examples of Professional Nursing Concepts Category With Associated Macroconcepts and Concepts**

Concept Category	Macro-Concept	Examples of Concepts
Professional Nursing Concepts	Holistic Care	Patient-Centered Care, Ethics, Diversity, Equity, Inclusion
	Health Care Infrastructures	Health Care Organizations, Health Care Economics, Health Policy, Health Care Law
	Personal Development	Professional Identity, Resilience, Leadership, Clinical Judgment
	Care Competencies	Communication, Collaboration, Quality & Safety, Health Equity, Population Health, Technology, and Informatics

TABLE 4.4 ■ **Examples of Health Care Recipient Concept Category With Associated Macroconcepts and Concepts**

Concept Category	Macro-Concept	Concepts
Health Care Recipient	Attributes	Development, Functional Ability, Family Dynamics, Genetics
	Personal Preferences	Culture, Spirituality, Motivation, Self-Management

Health care recipient concepts are considered from three contexts: the *individual*, the *family*, and the *community* (with community care ranging from a local to a global perspective). These contexts serve as guiding principles related to how the concepts are selected, presented, and applied (see Fig. 4.4). For example, the concept of *Culture* represents the shared attitudes, beliefs, traditions, norms, values, and preferences of individuals and groups of people. Culture should be considered when providing care to an individual health care recipient, and it should be considered in the context of that individual's family members—recognizing that there may be value conflict between the two. Culture from the perspective of community has application when doing work in public health nursing and when setting health policy. Context parameters such as these (the individual, family, and community) help with the selection process and provide clarity for use within the curriculum.

SELECTING AND IDENTIFYING CONCEPTS

Selecting concepts generally follows after (or in conjunction with) determining concept categories. Often, faculty will have ideas about certain concepts that should be included in a curriculum, and thus the formation of concept categories is helpful. One of the biggest challenges, however, is determining how many and which concepts to include. The hallmarks of "good" or well-chosen concepts to include in a nursing curriculum are presented in Box 4.1. Typically, the concepts should be very familiar and understandable to nursing faculty because they

---

BOX 4.1 ■ Hallmarks of Concepts for Nursing Education Curricula

- The concept represents an important group of conditions or situations (exemplars) encountered in nursing practice.
- The concept has application across multiple courses and contexts within the curriculum.
- The concept is helpful to the learner.
- The concept can be used logically and consistently by all faculty.

represent the scope of nursing practice. If there is a lot of confusion among faculty about a proposed concept, it should be critically analyzed to determine if it represents a concept associated with a specialty (a microconcept) or if it really represents a larger category of concepts (a macroconcept). Distinctions between microconcepts and macroconcepts are presented in Chapter 1.

Because concepts should reflect contemporary nursing and health care practice, an examination of the nursing and other health sciences literature is helpful. As one example (and mentioned previously), the American Association of Colleges of Nursing identified eight concepts and 10 domains (which are similar to concepts) in *The Essentials* (AACN, 2021); these would be a good starting point for consideration of inclusion into the curriculum. Another strategy is to review the list of concepts included in other concept-based curricula. A study involving a survey of 10 nursing programs or consortiums using a concept-based curriculum identified a total of 54 benchmark concepts—in other words, those that were most prevalent among reporting schools (Giddens et al., 2012). Another study reported results from a survey to validate concepts and exemplars used in concept-based curricula. The survey, developed by a 5-member task force and validated by 11 independent reviewers, included 47 concepts and 290 exemplars. A total of 68 respondents completed the survey, which led to 46 concepts and 245 exemplars being included in a final framework (Brussow et al., 2019). Both studies reveal that programs offering a concept-based curricula have similar featured concepts, and also confirm there is not a single "correct" list. In other words, one should expect some variability in the concepts if comparing concept-based curricula across several schools. Furthermore, the concepts included in a concept-based curriculum can and will evolve as healthcare changes.

As concepts are recommended and negotiated, a consistent, systematic selection process should be applied to determine whether a concept is "accepted" or "rejected" for final inclusion in a curriculum. Five questions that link back to the hallmarks of a "good" concept can be used to facilitate such a process:

1. Does the concept represent an important group of conditions or situations (exemplars) encountered in contemporary nursing practice?
2. Can the concept be applied across multiple courses and contexts within the curriculum?
3. Is the concept useful to the learner? In other words, will the learner find a clear application of the concept to the courses and clinical experiences?
4. Can the concept be used logically and consistently by all faculty?
5. Is the concept sustainable? In other words, is this a concept that will be applicable in years to come?

Another element associated with concept selection is clearly defining and developing the concept. As discussed in Chapter 3, faculty must have a shared understanding of the concept—how it is defined, what it represents, how it is applied, and how it will be taught. It is recommended that a template be followed so this work progresses consistently. The template may vary depending on the type of concept category because one template does not necessarily work for all categories. A sample template for health and illness concepts and a template that

---

BOX 4.2 ■ Sample Template for Health and Illness Concepts

- Definition
- Scope, type, or category(s)
- Individual risk factors and populations at risk
- Physiological process and consequences
- Assessment
  - History
  - Examination
  - Diagnostic studies
- Clinical management and Competencies
  - Primary prevention
  - Secondary prevention (screening)
  - Collaborative interventions
- Interrelated concepts

BOX 4.3 ■ Sample Template for Professional Nursing Concepts and Health Care Recipient Concepts

- Definition
- Scope, type, or categories
- Attributes
- Theoretical links
- Context to nursing and health care
- Interrelated concepts

---

works for professional nursing and health care recipient concepts are provided in Boxes 4.2 and 4.3, respectively. A more detailed discussion regarding concept development for a curriculum and teaching can be found in Chapter 3.

COMPETENCIES

A competency-based approach in health sciences education is becoming more prevalent (AACN, 2019; Kavanagh and Sharpnack, 2021; Lucey, 2018), and many nursing programs are following this trend by incorporating competencies into the curriculum. As discussed in Chapter 2, a competency is a general statement that describes the knowledge, skills, attitudes, and behaviors necessary for students to successfully perform in a professional context thus, they not only provide direction for teaching but are also used to assess students' progress while in a program.

The structure of a concept-based curriculum lends itself well to the use and application of competencies because competencies are written for each concept/domain. Because competencies describe what is expected of the learner at the end of the educational program, they provide direction for the teaching learning process and learner assessment. Competencies are developed in tandem with the concepts and should link clearly throughout the curriculum and to the program learning outcomes (see Table 4.1); multiple competencies link to the broad program outcomes (Sullivan, 2016). Because competency statements drive the assessment of student learning for the concepts, they also serve as an important component of program evaluation. A "backward design" approach is useful during curriculum development to optimize the clear links between concepts/competencies, teaching, and assessment. Backward design refers to the process of starting with the end point in mind (meaning the students' ability to demonstrate competency) and then develop teaching and learning strategies to ensure students have an opportunity to learn what is expected. Assessment strategies are developed to facilitate student progress toward competency attainment. The backward design concept is illustrated in Fig. 4.2. Competencies (which reflect the desired endpoint) are a component of concepts and domains, and these are established before the development of courses, teaching/learning strategies, and assessment. Courses and learning activities are developed with that endpoint in mind to ensure students can demonstrate competencies by the end of the program. Thus concepts, domains, and competencies are represented throughout the program curriculum as opposed to an isolated course.

Competency statements should be observable, measurable, and specific; they usually begin with an action verb. For example, a competency statement for Systems-Based Practice is "Coordinate patient care within the health care system relevant to one's clinical specialty" (Englander et al., 2013, p. 1092). Many national organizations have developed and published competencies and propose that competencies are incorporated into nursing curricula (AACN, 2021; Interprofessional Education Collaborative IPEC, 2016; QSEN, n.d.); thus, the adoption of published competency statements is an option if these match with concepts identified for the curriculum.

SELECTING EXEMPLARS

Exemplars provide a clinical context for the concept. Exemplars—or "examples"—are necessary for deep conceptual learning because they provide specific information, facts, topics, and situations representing the concept for the broader, more abstract concept. Conceptual learning holds limited value unless students can anchor what they have learned to specific examples. Exemplars are where traditional nursing content fits within a concept-based curriculum. The use of facts and base information is absolutely necessary as part of the conceptual learning process because facts support conceptual learning, and conceptual understanding supports the students' ability to make generalizations—thus higher-order cognitive thinking. For example, the student must understand facts associated with the heart and circulatory system as a foundation for learning the concept of perfusion. Furthermore, facts associated with exemplars (such as acute myocardial infarction) provide further opportunities to deepen the conceptual understanding associated with perfusion.

In a concept-based curriculum, exemplars are carefully selected to minimize excessive curricular content. It is not uncommon for nursing faculty to be initially skeptical about limiting the number of exemplars. The value of managing excessive curriculum content is based on the premise that when students gain a deep understanding of a concept, they are able to make connections from the concept to other exemplars—even ones they have not been formally taught in the classroom. It is also important to remember that students will be exposed to far more exemplars in the clinical setting when providing care to patients and families. Thus, an essential part of the concept-based curriculum is capitalizing on students' exposure to exemplars that are not formally taught in the didactic courses and helping students make purposeful cognitive connections.

Setting a process for exemplar selection helps to reduce the temptation to include exemplars that happen to be a favorite topic of one or more faculty, which tends to lead to a curriculum pitfall of excessive content. Ideally, data-driven decisions are made to select exemplars. When data-driven decisions are made, students will be exposed to the most important and prevalent content. In other words, the faculty will focus on the most common things the student will see in practice as it relates to that concept. Health and illness concepts are best selected based on state, national, and global health incidence and prevalence statistics (such as the Centers for Disease Control and Prevention). However, there may be an occasional situation where an exemplar is selected because it has a unique value in illustrating the concept. Exemplars for professional nursing concepts and health care recipient attributes are best identified by current literature and contemporary events, although some more historical events may have a particular value if they have forever influenced nursing and health care practice today. Subject matter experts provide another option for the selection of exemplars, as described by Brussow and colleagues (Brussow et al., 2019).

Another challenge when selecting exemplars is that most exemplars link to multiple concepts; thus, there is a risk of duplication of content within the curriculum. For example, the exemplar pneumonia logically links to *Infection, Gas Exchange, Fatigue,* and *Fluid and Electrolyte Balance*—but it is completely unnecessary to teach pneumonia four times as an exemplar of four different concepts! A curriculum plan or map that clearly shows exemplars used for each concept helps to minimize this issue. When teaching a specific exemplar, the lesson plan should include time for students to reflect on other concepts that are interrelated with the exemplar.

Course Design and Sequencing

Courses within a curriculum should reflect the program learning outcomes and should be logically sequenced to facilitate students' achievement of those program learning outcomes. Course sequencing refers to the order in which courses are taken by a student. Curriculum content should build over the academic program; thus, faculty must carefully consider not only content within a specific course, but also how courses collectively build on previous learning. If there is an especially important connection between one course that builds on another, a prerequisite requirement is often used. Course sequencing is communicated to students through a published *program of study* (also known as a plan of study), which outlines what courses should be taken and when. If a program offers full-time and part-time options, a program of study for each may be needed to show expected sequencing.

Expectations of student learning within courses are written as course learning outcomes and are used to guide course content, organization, learning, and assessment of student learning within the course. In a concept-based curriculum, course learning outcomes should clearly emphasize the application of concepts within the course and must link to the program learning outcomes. An example of a course learning outcome that might be developed within a concept-based curriculum (along with concepts and competencies) was presented earlier in this chapter (see Table 4.1). Notice the linkages between course learning outcomes, concepts, competencies, and program learning outcomes. More detail regarding writing learning outcomes is presented in Chapter 6.

Specific elements for course development include determining the type of course (e.g., lab, clinical, seminar, or didactic), the course description, student learning outcomes for the course, the number of academic credits, course delivery, a course outline (i.e., delineation of specific topics/content featured within the course), and planned strategies for teaching, learning, and evaluation. Teaching, learning, and evaluation strategies should align with the student learning outcomes and the type of course. Arrangement and sequencing of content within a course should be considered to ensure continuity, consistency, and balance.

There are many additional variables related to curriculum development that influence decisions about courses, course design, and sequencing. First, the type of degree offered drives the total number of credit hours; thus, the number of credits for nursing courses will vary. Also, the institution may influence some of the courses offered and the sequencing of those courses. The semester students are admitted to the nursing program (e.g., direct entry, entry after the first semester, entry after one year, or entry after two years) must also be considered. Finally, the prerequisites and corequisites influence what is considered primary content or review content. For example, if anatomy, physiology, and pathophysiology are prerequisite courses taken before entry into the nursing curriculum, the courses will look different than if the content from these courses (anatomy, physiology, and pathophysiology) are to be integrated into the nursing courses.

DIDACTIC COURSES

Another important decision must be made regarding how concepts will be applied within didactic courses. Two common paths may be taken: (1) integrated into traditional population-focused and topic-focused courses, or (2) concept-focused courses.

Integration Into Population-Focused and Topic-Focused Courses

For years, nursing curricula have arranged content around population (such as pediatric, maternal child, adult, and geriatrics) and topic areas (such as mental health, leadership, and community). When this approach is used for a concept-based curriculum, concepts are a common link between and among courses. For example, all the health and illness concepts apply to all population groups and thus are the core organizers of content for these courses. The focus of the concept presentation and exemplars are based on the population-specific elements for that concept. Professional nursing concepts fit into many of the fundamentals and leadership-type courses. In this approach, clinical courses continue to be closely linked to the traditional population-focused didactic courses.

One advantage to the population-focused and topic-focused approach is that many of the courses and clinical experiences maintain a level of familiarity and may be more readily accepted by faculty. A drawback to this approach is that faculty are tempted to change very little and claim they teach the concepts while continuing to overload students with content. Also, there is the potential for each faculty member in each course to teach the concept overview, which would result in duplication of effort.

MISCONCEPTIONS AND CLARIFICATIONS

Misconception: A simple way to develop a concept-based curriculum is to identify major concepts within courses of an existing curriculum.

Clarification: Designing a concept-based curriculum does not occur by simply identifying concepts in an existing curriculum, nor does it occur by adding concepts to an existing curriculum (i.e., an "add-on" approach). Concepts and competencies provide the structural framework for courses, content, and assessment. A *backward design* approach ensures that concepts and related competencies drive course redesign with a specific plan for integrating concepts within the courses.

Concept-Focused Courses

Another approach is to develop concept-focused courses that feature integration of population groups. Courses may follow the identified concept categories (Table 4.5). For example, there may be a series of courses that feature health and illness concepts, a series of courses that feature professional nursing concepts, and a course that features health care recipient concepts. If macroconcepts are identified within concept categories, these may also be useful to consider so that concepts that are closely related are taught in a similar course.

When a concept-focused course approach is used, concepts and dedicated exemplars are featured once in the designated didactic course. Thereafter the concepts are presented as interrelated concepts. Conceptual links across population groups and types of settings are made. Clinical courses should be designed to follow concept courses and apply concepts from *all* courses (health and illness, professional nursing concepts, and health care recipient concepts) into the clinical experience. In other words, clinical education represents the application and synthesis of all concepts, not just one group of concepts, in a variety of clinical sites and working with a variety of patient populations.

TABLE 4.5 ■ Sample of Course Arrangement in a Concept-Based Curriculum for a Four-Semester Nursing Program (Upper Division)

SEMESTER 1	SEMESTER 2
Nursing Skills and Assessment Lab	Health and Illness Concepts II
Patient Attributes Concepts	Professional Nursing Concepts I
Health and Illness Concepts I	Evidence-Based Nursing Practice
Clinical Practicum I	Clinical Practicum II
SEMESTER 3	**SEMESTER 4**
Health and Illness Concepts III	Global Health
Professional Nursing Concepts II	Concept Synthesis
Clinical Practicum III	Clinical Practicum V
Clinical Practicum IV	Capstone

The benefit to this approach is that the concept is presented in greater depth, allowing for a deeper understanding to occur through exemplar reinforcement. However, this approach is not without challenges. It requires a very different teaching expectation among faculty and may result in the need for team teaching in the didactic courses. For example, the concept of *Gas Exchange* may be easy enough to teach, but the exemplars are likely to be representative of the health conditions across the age span, such as asthma in children and pneumonia in older adults. This approach also deemphasizes specialty content, and thus it is important that students have varied clinical experiences so they have clinical exposure across populations and specialties.

In addition to concept-featured courses, consideration of other types of courses should be included. As an example, a fundamentals course that teaches basic nursing skills and health assessment skills may still be necessary. In a baccalaureate curriculum, faculty may wish to offer a separate course focusing on community-based nursing, public health nursing, or nursing research. When this is the case, applicable core concepts are still to be woven into these courses.

CLINICAL COURSES

Decisions about the design of clinical courses are just as important as didactic course decisions. Furthermore, specific clinical learning activities (including simulation) should be incorporated into the overall curriculum plan. The conceptual approach offers an opportunity to break away from the traditional clinical education model that has been in place for well over 50 years. The emphasis has historically been placed on inpatient clinical courses that focus on caring for an assigned patient or patients, mimicking the work assignments of staff nurses in a designated clinical focus area. Students typically go to the unit to meet their assigned patient, review the medical record and prepare required clinical paperwork before their clinical experience. During the clinical day, students receive, report, and care for their assigned patient(s), which may include the following activities: hygiene care, toileting, activity and exercise patient assessment, nutrition, and dietary needs, medication administration, and a number of other interventions. For many care activities, direct supervision by the nursing instructor or a primary nurse is required. Throughout the program, the advancement of clinical expertise is measured by the number and complexity of the patients assigned and the gradual increase in independence demonstrated by the student in the provision of care. Although the "patient of the day" approach still holds value, there are some clear downsides, including a tendency for students to focus on tasks and considerable downtime experienced by students as they wait for the necessary supervision (by an instructor or primary nurse) to complete nursing intervention (such as a dressing change or administering a medication). This type of clinical learning should be considered one teaching strategy among many other strategies used for clinical education.

Clinical courses designed for a concept-based curriculum include a variety of learning opportunities for students to apply several concepts in a number of ways and in a number of clinical situations with an intentional emphasis on opportunities to demonstrate achievement of related competencies. Clinical courses should link to didactic courses in that the application of concepts from didactic courses should be emphasized. The learning activities can vary from the standard "patient of the day" assignment to a multitude of "concept-focused" learning within the clinical area, with the emphasis on repeated opportunities to learn for competency attainment. For example, students might be assigned to study the concepts of *Immunity, Inflammation,* and *Infection* within a designated group of patients and also consider how the concepts of *Health Policy* and *Health Care Economics* apply to the patient situations. Learning could focus on comparing and contrasting evidence of the positive or ineffective immune status and evidence of, or risk for, inflammation and infection (among multiple patients) and includes the reinforcement of previously learned or new exemplars representing those concepts. Students might be asked to review policies that impact the care and compare health payment plans of the patients they are caring for. Simulation, with an emphasis on specified concepts and competencies, is another type of clinical learning activity that is effective. Further examples of concept-based teaching strategies for clinical education are presented in Chapter 7.

Clinical experiences with a variety of population groups and settings (e.g., pediatrics, adults, geriatrics, mental health, intensive care, and community) are needed, but with less emphasis placed on attempting to get the exact same set of clinical experiences for all students. For example, in some programs offering a concept-based curriculum, students have an opportunity to choose the clinical courses (known as clinical intensives) that appeal to them after completing foundational clinical courses. Thus, in a given semester, students in the same cohort are applying concepts from the didactic concept courses in different clinical areas. Such an approach allows greater flexibility and efficiency in the way clinical sites are used (Giddens et al., 2008).

Program Evaluation

Program evaluation is a process that assesses program effectiveness through the evaluation of program learning outcomes, competencies, and other standardized program metrics required by certification and regulatory bodies. There has been an increased emphasis on the intentional measurement of program learning outcomes in higher education—this in response to the public's expectation for accountability (Boland, 2004). Program evaluation is planned as a part of curriculum development and continues during and after implementation.

Program learning outcomes, competencies, and course level learning outcomes provide the infrastructure for an evaluation plan. A strong evaluation plan involves having a clear understanding of the evaluation standards and type of data to collect with a consistent and continuous data collection process using a variety of data collection methods. Aggregate-level data are collected at the course level, predetermined markers along the way, at the end of the program, and after graduation. Data sources include people (students, alumni, faculty, employers, preceptors, nurses), program reports, curriculum and course documents, evaluation tools, and agency reports. A clear plan for regular data analysis and reporting is needed so that data are used to inform curricular improvements.

LICENSURE PASS RATES

One of the most recognized and visible measures of program effectiveness and quality for prelicensure nursing programs is first-time pass rates on the National Council Licensure Examination for Registered Nurses (NCLEX). A review of the detailed NCLEX test plan reveals the bulk of the test plan is based on concepts; thus, a concept-based curriculum is a practical way to prepare graduates. All state Boards of Nursing and all three nursing accreditation bodies require a specific passing rate. Both the Accreditation Commission for Education in Nursing (ACEN) and the Commission on Collegiate Nursing Education (CCNE) guidelines require schools to achieve 80% first-time pass rates (Accreditation Commission for Education in Nursing [ACEN], 2021; Commission on Collegiate Nursing Education [CCNE], 2018).

When analyzing NCLEX pass rates, faculty should consider more than the annual pass rate to determine if the program is providing the education needed to earn a passing score on the examination. The National Council of State Boards of Nursing has a service available that provides each nursing program with a specific program report. These reports are important because they reflect actual performance on the NCLEX and provide a wealth of information about the scores of the school's graduates in specific areas of the curriculum compared with graduates from other programs. The specific areas align with many of the concepts in a concept-based curriculum. For example, the reports include the graduates' achievement in areas such as nutrition; elimination; comfort, rest, activity, and mobility; growth and development; and immunity, as well as many other areas that align with curricular concepts. NCLEX Program Reports are published twice a year, allowing faculty to monitor data trends over a number of reporting periods to identify areas that are consistently weak and for which curriculum changes should be considered.

PROGRAM COMPLETION RATES

A common metric included in a program evaluation plan is program completion rates. Completion rates reflect the percentage of students who successfully complete the program in a designated timeframe. Nursing accreditation agencies consider completion rates as a key quality indicator. As one example, the CCNE guidelines require schools to have a 70% completion rate (CCNE, 2018).

EMPLOYMENT RATES

Another common metric measured in the program evaluation plan is the employment rates of graduates. These data are often collected at graduation time (as part of an exit survey) or after graduation as part of an alumni survey. Employment rates are particularly of interest to institutional and nursing accreditation bodies because of the issue of student debt and the ability of a student to repay school loans. As an example, the CCNE guidelines require schools to demonstrate employment rates at 70% or higher (CCNE, 2018).

AGGREGATE ASSESSMENT OF STUDENT LEARNING

Most colleges and universities have a system-wide process to assess learning outcomes annually. A typical plan involves determining specific assessment measures with metrics/targets for an academic year. This process is applied to any curriculum (including a concept-based curriculum). Examples of data collected could include papers, examinations, rubrics, or projects that provide evidence of student attainment of selected outcomes—and typically link to a concept or competency. In many colleges and universities there is a centralized place and process where data are entered into a database which then allows for the generation of aggregate outcomes reported on a predetermined timeframe (typically, these reports reflect an academic year).

AGGREGATE COURSE EVALUATIONS

Feedback from students about the effectiveness of courses in helping them achieve the course learning outcomes is imperative for ongoing program improvement. The completion of course evaluations by students is a well-established practice in education and should also be used in the concept-based curriculum. Of major importance is the students' evaluation of whether the course learning activities provided the opportunity to meet the course learning outcomes and learn the concepts presented in the course. Specific to conceptual learning, potential questions that could be incorporated into course evaluations could include:

1. Did the teaching strategies engage you in activities to develop a thorough understanding of the concepts addressed in the course?
2. Did the teaching strategies provide ample opportunity to apply concepts to nursing and patient situations in the classroom or clinical setting?
3. Were there ample opportunities for feedback related to associated competencies?

AGGREGATE PROGRAM SATISFACTION

The satisfaction a program among graduates is another important indicator of a quality program. An end-of-program survey, sent to students near the time of graduation, provides an opportunity to assess a number of variables important to faculty. Two common measures include overall satisfaction with the program and perceptions regarding the adequacy of preparation. A similar survey may be sent to graduates 1 to 3 years after program completion to determine if their perceptions have changed as a result of being out in clinical practice. That is, graduates should be asked how well they can perform the behaviors and characteristics that are indicative of the program learning outcomes and if they have encountered any job responsibilities they are expected to perform frequently that they were not prepared to perform.

Tips for Success: Developing and Implementing the Concept-Based Curriculum

Most faculty are aware of the significant effort associated with developing and implementing a new curriculum, and barriers to implementation of a concept-based curriculum have been reported by many. A recent survey involving a convenience sample of faculty and administrators in schools adopting a concept-based curriculum reported on reasons for adoption and challenges experienced by faculty (Sportsman and Pleasant, 2017). Survey results revealed the most reported reason for change to a concept-based curriculum was driven by faculty themselves—36% of respondents indicated that faculty initiated the change. However, this also suggests that for many, other variables were responsible for the change. The most reported challenge, found by the researchers, was the lack of faculty education regarding a concept-based curriculum.

In a review of the literature regarding concept-based curriculum implementation, Repsha and colleagues confirmed that the most commonly reported challenges include faculty lacking understanding of concept-based curriculum, a lack of agreement on concepts to include in the curriculum, concerns related to teaching, and fear of the unknown—and concern for a potential drop in first-time NCLEX-RN pass rates (Repsha et al., 2020).

The following sections offer tips to overcome barriers and enhance success.

BUILD SUPPORT FOR CRITICAL MASS

The reaction and emotions expressed among faculty will range from being thrilled about the change to anger. Some faculty members who do not understand the conceptual approach may not fully engage in the curriculum process, and others may continually voice concerns. Occasionally a faculty member may even be overtly disruptive to work. When this occurs, supporting faculty may become discouraged. They may also worry about not gaining full consensus among the faculty. Although full consensus is ideal, in most cases, it is unrealistic. Building support for the concept-based curriculum among faculty often occurs over time. As more faculty understand, the curriculum work will eventually reach a *critical mass* of support to move forward. Energy should be directed toward working with those who seek change.

MANAGING RESISTANCE

Any new curriculum (especially a concept-based curriculum) represents a significant effort from the curriculum committee and faculty assigned to teach new courses. This can be threatening because some nurse educators may be forced to step out of their comfort zones—meaning they will be asked to teach differently. Resistance to change is a natural reaction (mainly when the proposed change is not universally or well understood). Anticipating and accepting resistance as a normal part of the process is helpful so that strategies can be developed to ensure forward movement. Resistance is usually put forth by one or more strongly vested faculty who defend the old curriculum. Common arguments against change (presented below) can be easily countered by using non-adversarial responses.

"We Have Always Done It This Way! Why Should We Change?"

Extensive changes in health care, coupled with a growing call for change, make this argument easy to address. Two early reports from the Institute of Medicine (IOM), *Crossing the Quality Chasm* (IOM, 2001) and *Health Professions Education* (IOM, 2003), called for improvements to be made in health sciences education to improve the quality of care. Specifically, several competencies such as patient-centered care, evidence-based medicine, working as part of an interdisciplinary team, focusing on quality improvement, and using information technology were emphasized, along with the need to address changing student demographics and teaching using active learning strategies (IOM, 2003). Another landmark publication, *Educating Nurses* (Benner et al., 2010), also describes the need for a radical transformation of the education of nurses. A focus on and delivery of content in the traditional way does little to prepare nurses for the "situated cognition and action" needed for clinical practice (Benner et al., 2010, p. 13). More recently, the *Future of Nursing: 2020–2030* called for the need for substantial change by stating, "To change nursing education meaningfully so as to produce nurses who are prepared to meet the challenges in the decade ahead, will require changes in four areas: what is taught, how it is taught, who the students are, and who teaches them" (National Academies of Sciences, Engineering, and Medicine [NASEM], 2021, p. 190). This statement is truly profound! Although these reports do not specify that a conceptual approach is needed, all emphasize the need for an improved education system for effective health care delivery. In other words, the traditional approach to nursing education is outdated and is no longer preparing nurses adequately for the current health care system. It is simply the professional and ethical obligation of a higher-education professional to address and embrace this call for critical change within the nursing profession.

"Our NCLEX Pass Rates Are Good"

One of the biggest barriers to innovative curriculum work is the justifiable fear of reduced first-time pass rates on the National Council Licensure Examination (NCLEX). For years, first-time NCLEX pass rates have unofficially served as the gold standard measure of the quality of a nursing program. The Boards of Nursing in all states closely monitor first-time pass rates, setting a minimum standard expected of schools—which in some cases may create additional concern. In truth, the first-time NCLEX pass rate is only one indicator of program quality considered by accreditors. Other important measures include student and program measures. Examples of student measures include evidence of achievement of program outcomes, competencies, and student learning outcomes within courses, time to graduation, graduation rates, and the diversity of student enrollment. Program measures include an adequate number of qualified full-time faculty for the program(s) offered; tracking, orientation, and evaluation of preceptors and adjunct faculty; integrity of the curriculum; and a systematic approach to curriculum evaluation. The point is, a nursing program can have excellent first-time pass rates and yet can fail to address the changing needs of the nursing workforce. There is no intent to suggest that concept-based curricula will increase first-time pass rates, but no evidence exists that programs with a concept-based curriculum have a lower pass rate. In a survey of 57 nursing programs offering a concept-based curriculum, 35% reported higher first-time pass rates, 42% reported no changes in first-time pass rates, and 5% reported lower first-time pass rates. Eighteen percent of respondents did not know the impact on first-time pass rates (many had not yet graduated students from their new concept-based curriculum (Sportsman, 2014).

Additionally, there have been five published studies in the nursing literature that have specifically reported NCLEX pass rates after implementing a concept-based curriculum. In four of the five studies, no significant change in NCLEX pass rates was reported (Duncan and Schultz, 2015; Lewis, 2014; Murray et al., 2015; and Patterson et al., 2016). One published study (Giddens and Morton, 2010) reported a drop in NCLEX pass rates with the first graduating cohort, but with a return to pre-curriculum change pass rates in subsequent cohorts. A recent review of the literature by Repsha et al. (2020) reported no differences in first-time NCLEX pass rates among schools adopting a conceptual approach.

"What Evidence Proves the Conceptual Approach Is Better?"

Interestingly, this question is raised over and over again, especially when there is plenty of evidence that our traditional approaches to educating the healthcare workforce have not been effective in the changing healthcare environment (Benner et al., 2010; IOM, 2001, 2003; Kavanagh and Sharpnack, 2021; National Academies of Sciences, Engineering, and Medicine [NASEM], 2021).

One can defend the traditional approach by citing "evidence" based on first-time NCLEX pass rates, as though this is the only evidence that counts, but, as noted above, this argument does not hold. Although there is no "proof" that a conceptual approach to nursing education is better, the education discipline has plenty of evidence regarding improvements in learning and improvements in content management when the conceptual approach is applied (Ambrose et al., 2010; Erikson, 2008; Schmidt et al., 1997; Sousa, 2010; Zull, 2002). Over time, as more nurse educators adopt the conceptual approach, we can expect the availability of published programs and student learning outcomes.

"Our Faculty Workloads Are Too Heavy"

The nationwide faculty shortage and the recent pandemic have had several implications for nursing programs, but what is especially problematic is the effect on faculty work assignments. It is unlikely that any nursing program has faculty who are not concerned about the amount of work associated with their jobs. Thus, this is a statement and argument that is universally heard with any project, initiative, or change introduced to faculty groups. It is true that adopting the conceptual approach requires significant effort initially—not only with curriculum development but also to change teaching. However, over time faculty learn how to teach conceptually effectively, and often they find that the teaching effort is more effective and efficient.

An expectation of all faculty, regardless of the type of institution or type of discipline, is maintaining currency in educational delivery. Curriculum development and advancing one's teaching should not be presented as an "add-on" or "additional work"—rather, this should be presented as a professional obligation to the students, institution, and profession. Furthermore, once the curriculum is developed and faculty begin the process of transitioning their teaching practice, there is often a level of energy and excitement that is associated with the teaching-learning process.

SECURE RESOURCES

Undertaking any major effort is met with greater acceptance if adequate resources are available. Examples of helpful resources include:

- Expert consultation from nursing faculty experienced in the development of a concept-based curriculum or consultation from faculty in other disciplines, such as education
- Site visits to nursing programs that have successfully adopted a concept-based curriculum
- A dedicated work assignment for key faculty who are leading the curriculum change
- Faculty development opportunities, especially in the area of concept-based teaching and learning
- Support from senior administrators in the nursing program, particularly for additional help needed or flexibility in teaching assignments, admissions, and course scheduling as the new curriculum is rolled out.

In addition to the above-mentioned strategies for curriculum development, Sportsman and Pleasant (2017) reported that faculty development for teaching and learning was the most significant support needed to implement a concept-based curriculum.

EXPECT HARD WORK AND ENCOURAGE AND SUPPORT ONE ANOTHER

Curriculum redesign is very challenging work that takes a great deal of time. Faculty should not begin with an expectation that the process will be completed quickly. A great deal of discussion, negotiating, and reflection is needed at the beginning of the process to elicit input and build the initial support needed to begin work, let alone the numerous meetings and work needed for the actual curriculum design. Developing a trusting, encouraging, and supportive relationship among the faculty—particularly those directly involved in the curriculum work—helps to sustain the effort needed over time.

ENGAGE CLINICAL PARTNERS

One of the most important things faculty can and should do as part of the curriculum redesign process is to collaborate with nurses in clinical practice settings (particularly those from clinical agencies where students complete clinical experiences). The perspective of clinicians in practice provides important input, will enrich the work, and deepen the relationships between the nursing school and the clinical agency. Eliciting input and support from these important stakeholders as part of the curriculum development process will also facilitate acceptance of the planned changes. This is particularly important when redesigning clinical education and attempting to implement significantly different learning activities within the various clinical sites.

Summary

This chapter has reviewed the general steps associated with the development of a concept-based curriculum. The general curriculum development process for a concept-based curriculum is the same as any curriculum process; what is unique is the curriculum design and the incorporation of concepts and competencies. The didactic and clinical course design and teaching practices will support the conceptual design and intent of the curriculum. Concepts used for the curriculum represent concepts of nursing practice as opposed to concepts representing the discipline of nursing from a theoretical perspective. An advantage of a concept-based curriculum is to minimize content by carefully considering the concepts and the number of exemplars to include in the curriculum. Consideration for evaluating student learning and the program evaluation plan is planned as part of the curriculum design. Finally, the curriculum development and revision process is difficult. Faculty often feel unprepared to do this work, and resistance among faculty may occur. Resistance is not a reason to abandon the idea but rather represents a difference in the values and perspectives of faculty. The lack of understanding related to the conceptual approach is often the greatest source of resistance.

References

Accreditation Commission for Education in Nursing (ACEN). *ACEN Accreditation Manual 2017 Standards and Criteria.* Atlanta GA: ACEN; 2021.

American Association of Colleges of Nursing (AACN). *AACN's vision for academic nursing. AACN;* 2019. https://www.aacnnursing.org/Portals/42/News/White-Papers/Vision-Academic-Nursing.pdf.

American Association of Colleges of Nursing (AACN). *The Essentials: Core Competencies for Professional Nursing Education. AACN;* 2021. https://www.aacnnursing.org/Portals/42/AcademicNursing/pdf/Essentials-2021.pdf.

Ambrose SA, Bridges MW, DiPietro M, et al. *How Learning Works. 7 Research-Based Principles for Smart Teaching.* San Francisco, CA: John Wiley & Sons; 2010.

Benner P, Sutphen M, Leonard V, et al. *Educating Nurses: A Call for Radical Transformation.* San Francisco, CA: Josey-Bass; 2010.

Boland DL. Developing curriculum: frameworks, outcomes and competencies. In: Billings D, Halstead J, eds. *Teaching in Nursing.* 4th ed. St. Louis, MO: Elsevier; 2012.

Boland DL. Program evaluation and public accountability. In: Oermann M, Heinrich K, eds. *Annual Review of Nursing Education.* New York, NY: Springer; 2004.

Brussow JA, Roberts K, Scaruto M, et al. Concept-based curricula. A national study of critical concepts. *Nurse Educ.* 2019;44(1):15–19. https://doi.org/10.1097/NNE.0000000000000515.

Commission on Collegiate Nursing Education (CCNE). *Standards for Accreditation of Baccalaureate and Graduate Nursing Programs. CCNE;* 2018. https://www.aacnnursing.org/Portals/42/CCNE/PDF/Standards-Final-2018.pdf.

Csokasy J. A congruent curriculum: philosophical integrity from philosophy to outcomes. *J Nurs Educ.* 2002;41:469–470.

Duncan K, Schulz PS. Impact of change to a concept-based baccalaureate nursing curriculum on student and program outcomes. *J Nurs Educ.* 2015;54(3):S16–S20.

Englander R, Cameron T, Ballard AJ, et al. Toward a common taxonomy of competency domains for the health professions and competencies for physicians. *Acad Med.* 2013;88:1088–1094.

Erikson L. *Stirring the Head, Heart, and Soul: Redefining Curriculum, Instruction, and Concept-Based Learning.* Thousand Oaks, CA: Corwin Press; 2008.

Giddens J, Brady D, Brown P, et al. A new curriculum for a new era of nursing education. *Nurs Educ Perspect.* 2008;29:200–204.

Giddens J, Morton N. Report card: an evaluation of a concept-based curriculum. *Nurs Educ Perspect.* 2010;31:372–377.

Giddens J, Wright M, Gray I. Selecting concepts for a concept-based curriculum: application of a benchmark approach. *J Nurs Educ.* 2012;51:511–515.

Haydon JK, Smiley RA, Alexander M, et al. The NCSBN national simulation study: a longitudinal randomized, controlled study replacing clinical hours with simulation in prelicensure nursing education. *J Nurs Regul.* 2014;5(2):S1–S64.

Hopkins K, Kroning M. Leadership's role in curriculum revision. *Teach Learn Nurs.* 2021;16:166–168. https://doi.org/10.1016/j.teln.2020.11.002.

Institute of Medicine (IOM). *Crossing the Quality Chasm.* Washington, DC: National Academies Press; 2001.

Institute of Medicine (IOM). *Health Professions Education.* Washington, DC: National Academies Press; 2003.

Interprofessional Education Collaborative (IPEC). *Core Competencies for Interprofessional Collaborative Practice: 2016 Update.* Washington, DC: Interprofessional Education Collaborative; 2016.

INACSL Standards Committee. INASCL standards of best practice: Simulation^SM. *Clin Simul Nurs.* 2016;12:S5–S50. https://doi.org/10.1016/j.ecns.2016.10.001.

Josiah Macy Foundation. Registered Nurses: Partners in Transforming Primary Care. *Josiah Macy Foundation;* 2016. https://macyfoundation.org./publications/conference-summary-registered-nurses-partners-in-transforming-primary-care.

Kavanagh JM, Sharpnack PA. Crisis in competency: A defining moment in nursing education. *Online J Issues Nurs.* 2021;26(1).

Lewis L. Outcomes of a concept-based curriculum. *Teach Learn Nurs.* 2014;9:75–79.

Lucey CR. Achieving competency-based, time-variable health professions education. In: *Proceedings of a Conference Sponsored by Josiah Macy Jr. Foundation in June 2017.* New York, NY: Josiah Macy Jr. Foundation; 2018:2018. https://macyfoundation.org/assets/reports/publications/macy_monograph_2017_final.pdf.

Murray S, Laurent K, Gontarz J. Evaluation of a concept-based curriculum: a tool and process. *Teach Learn Nurs.* 2015;10:169–175.

National Academies of Sciences, Engineering, and Medicine (NASEM). *The Future of Nursing 2020–2030: Charting a Path to Achieve Health Equity.* Washington, DC: The National Academies Press; 2021. https://doi.org/10.17226/25982.

Ortiz MR. Patient-centered care: nursing knowledge and policy. *Nurs Sci Q.* 2018;21(3):291–295.

Patterson LD, Crager JM, Farmer A, et al. A strategy to ensure faculty engagement when assessing a concept-based curriculum. *J Nurs Educ.* 2016;55:467–470.

Quality and Safety Education in Nursing [QSEN] competencies, QSEN, n.d: Retrieved from: https://www.qsen.org/.

Repsha CL, Quinn BL, Peters AB. Implementing a concept-based nursing curriculum: a review of the literature. *Teach Learn Nurs.* 2020;15:66–71. https://doi.org/10.1016/j.teln.2019.09.006.

Schmidt WH, McKnight CC, Raizen S. *A Splintered Vision: An Investigation of U.S. Science and Mathematics Education, U.S. National Research Center for the Third International Mathematics and Science Study (TIMSS).* Dordrecht, Netherlands: Kluwer Academic Publishers; 1997.

Sousa DA. *Mind, Brain, and Education. Neuroscience Implications for the Classroom.* Bloomington, IL: Solution Tree Press; 2010.

Sportsman S. *Concept Based Curriculum in Nursing: Perceptions of the Trend.* Washington, DC: Academic Consulting Group. Elsevier; 2014.

Sportsman S, Pleasant T. Concept-based curricula: state of the innovation. *Teach Learn Nurs.* 2017;12:195–200.

Sullivan DT. An introduction to curriculum development. In: Billings D, Halstead J, eds. *Teaching in Nursing.* 5th ed. St. Louis, MO: Elsevier; 2016.

Whittmann-Price RA, Fasolka BJ. Objectives and outcomes: the fundamental difference. *Nurs Educ Perspect.* 2010;31:233–236.

Zull JE. *The Art of the Changing Brain.* Sterling, VA: Stylus Publishing; 2002.

CHAPTER 5

Conceptual Learning

A key challenge shared among all instructors—regardless of the discipline or student level—is creating an optimal platform for learning. In higher education, faculty are primarily hired because of expertise in their respective discipline and often lack an understanding of how people learn. Faculty tend to focus on honing a teaching style that works well for them, with little thought on how student learning occurs as a result of their efforts. A common assumption held by faculty is that students learn as a result of attending a class or completing a course. The flaw in this thinking is nested in a general lack of understanding about what learning is and the science behind learning. The truth is, learning is not something that is "done" to students by instructors; rather, learning is something that students accomplish themselves. Instructors have a role in facilitating this process by creating purposeful and engaging learning activities in an optimal learning environment.

Conceptual learning was identified in Chapter 1 as one of several separate but interrelated elements associated with the conceptual approach. The desired outcome associated with conceptual learning is that students gain a deep understanding of concepts and the ability to transfer ideas to other situations through cognitive connections. Nurse educators adopting the conceptual approach are usually eager to learn how to teach conceptually. However, gaining an understanding of the science of learning is foundational to teaching. Put another way, the science of instruction builds on the science of learning. Having an understanding about how learning occurs must precede conversations about best teaching practices. In this chapter, principles associated with the science of learning will be presented, along with the linkages to the conceptual approach.

Definition of Learning

There are many definitions of learning representing a wide range of perspectives. Ambrose and colleagues offer a contemporary definition reflective of the science of learning. They define learning as "a *process* that leads to *change* which occurs as a result of *experience* and increases the potential for improved performance and future learning" (Ambrose et al., 2010, p. 3). Emphasis on the words "process," "change," and "experience" represents three key components of the definition. *Process* is emphasized because learning is a brain-based physiological process that occurs in the mind. Learning cannot be directly seen or measured, but inferences that learning has occurred are made based on student performance. *Change* is emphasized because learning results in a change in students' knowledge, beliefs, behaviors, attitudes, and values. Although the change occurs over time, an enduring impact occurs. *Experience* is emphasized because learning is shaped by the interpretation and response to former and current experiences. Experiences take on many forms, some more powerful than others. In any given situation, students may or may not be aware of the influence of experiences on their learning. These key components become clearer in the sections that follow. How learning actually occurs has been debated for years, and, as a result, multiple classic learning theories have been proposed, including behaviorist, cognitivism, constructivism, cognitive development, and humanism. During the past few decades, there has been increasing interest in neuroscience and brain-based learning theories, grounded in the premise that biologic changes in the brain occur in response to learning. The intent of this chapter is not to present learning theories but rather to use neuroscience and brain-based theory to explain conceptual learning.

Educational Neuroscience: How the Brain Learns

Although the majority of brain development occurs during the prenatal period through early childhood, the brain continues to develop, adapt, and change in response to learning throughout life. Learning is a complex process with multiple variables. *Educational neuroscience* is a term used to describe the interrelationship between neuroscience, teaching practices (pedagogy), and psychology as key components of the learning process (Fig. 5.1). Essentially, the premise of

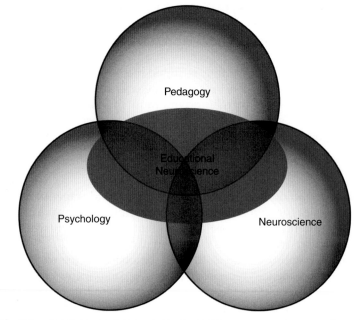

Fig. 5.1   Educational neuroscience represents pedagogy, neuroscience, and psychology.

educational neuroscience is that learning involves physiological changes within the brain (primarily through changes in neural circuitry); and the learning environment, instruction methods, and psychological factors of the learner influence the learning process. A significant focus of educational neuroscience is on the optimal conditions for the brain to learn (Ambrose et al., 2010; Connell, 2009; Jensen, 2008; Sosa, 2010). Learning is optimal when the brain is in a calm state, when the active learning is challenging (but not threatening), when multiple experiences are provided in a realistic context, and when the learner is required to connect previous knowledge to new knowledge.

It is imperative that all educators gain an understanding of these components to fully grasp how to effectively facilitate conceptual learning. In the sections that follow, a very brief review of brain structures and function is included as a foundation for understanding the process of learning. This discussion of brain function is only done with the intent to explain how the brain learns.

GENERAL BRAIN FUNCTION

A very simplistic summarization of what the brain does can be described in three words: *sensing*, *integrating*, and *responding*. **Sensing** refers to an ongoing process whereby the brain takes in data signals (input) from a variety of internal (physiological) and external (environmental) sources. The brain interfaces with millions of data signals, most of which do not require conscious thought. **Integrating** is the process of sorting and grouping data and then making sense of those data. Data sorting occurs immediately and does not require purposeful thought. Put another way, integration is the process of brain recognition and interpretation that occurs with the sum of all the data signals (Zull, 2002). **Responding** refers to the outcome of the data integration. Based on the sorting and grouping of data signals, the brain sends information to target areas, triggering a wide variety of physiological responses, including regulatory and motor responses (voluntary and automatic movements). The transfer of data signals—from sensory input, integration, to response—is continuous, cyclic, and automatic; sensory input triggers integrative activity, which activates physiological, cognitive, and motor responses (Fig. 5.2).

Brain Structures

The brain is a highly complex structure within the central nervous system and is composed of two major units: the cerebrum (also known as the telencephalon) and the brainstem.

Cerebrum. The cerebrum comprises the largest part of the human brain and is divided into two hemispheres (right and left), each of which are divided into four lobes (frontal, temporal, parietal, and occipital) as shown in Fig. 5.3. A general description of the four lobes is presented in Table 5.1. The outer layer covering the cerebrum is the cortex; together, these are referred to as the *cerebral cortex*. Neurons within the cortex are responsible for many of the highly sophisticated aspects of cognitive functioning. The cerebrum also contains two important

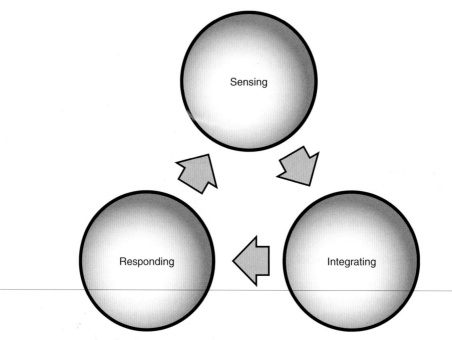

Fig. 5.2 Sensing, integrating, and responding are ongoing and continuous processes within the brain.

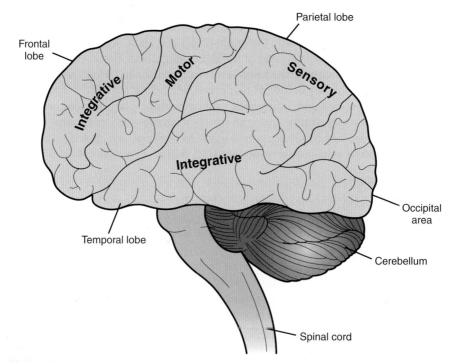

Fig. 5.3 Structures of the outer brain and functional areas for sensory, integrative, and motor functions.

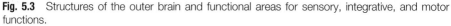

TABLE 5.1 ■ **Four Lobes of the Cerebral Cortex**

Lobe	Anatomical Facts	Functions
Frontal lobe	Five functional zones: primary motor cortex, premotor cortex, prefrontal cortex, medial frontal cortex, and anterior cingulate cortex.	Executive functions; problem solving, evaluation and hypothesis testing; responses to environmental cues; responses to internal information; behavior based on temporal memory; decision making for emotion and reward; behavior associated with context.
Parietal lobe	Anterior parietal lobe and posterior parietal cortex.	Guiding limb movements and manipulation of objects, visuospatial functions, spatial cognition. Coactive with other brain regions.
Temporal lobe	Five anatomic zones for auditory, visual, olfactory, emotional, and spatial processing.	Processes auditory and visual information; object recognition; spatial navigation, cognitive processes.
Occipital lobe	Occipital lobe tissues merge with temporal and parietal lobes, thus there are no clear boundaries.	Initiation of visual processing, perceiving form, movement, color

subcortical structures: the basal ganglia and the limbic system. Basal ganglia serve as a circuit with the cerebral cortex to connect sensory regions of the cortex to motor regions of the cortex to regulate movement and coordinate sensory and motor function. Sitting just above the brainstem, the limbic system is a group of structures that connect higher and lower brain functions (Fig. 5.4). Together these structures regulate emotion, mood, pleasure, and motivation, playing an important role in many behaviors considered conscious acts (Kolb and Whishaw, 2021). Box 5.1 presents a review of limbic structure functions.

Brainstem. The brainstem, located at the base of the brain, includes the hindbrain (cerebellum, medulla, pons, and reticular formation) midbrain, and diencephalon. The cerebellum, which protrudes above the brainstem core and beneath the occipital lobe of the cerebrum, coordinates movement and equilibrium (see Fig. 5.3). The diencephalon (which means *between brain*) includes the thalamic structures—hypothalamus, epithalamus, and thalamus. The thalamus is a relay center and transfers nearly all signals to the cerebral cortex. The hypothalamus regulates the autonomic nervous system and the endocrine system. Important to note, there is some controversy regarding the "status" of the diencephalon from an anatomical perspective. Because it borders the upper and lower part of the brain, some textbooks and other references place the thalamic structures as part of the forebrain within the limbic system, whereas others incorporate it as part of the brainstem. This variation and inconsistency can cause

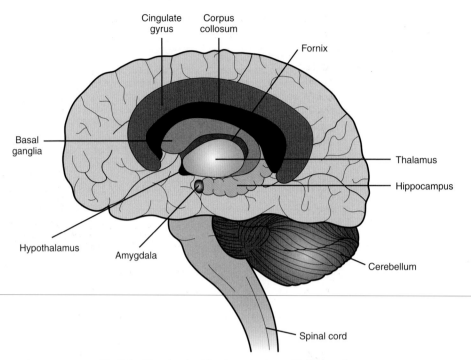

Fig. 5.4   Structures of the inner brain and limbic system.

BOX 5.1 ▪ Limbic Structure Functions

- The *amygdala* is a walnut-sized structure that influences the emotional states on sensory input and has a role in determining what memories retained. This structure has tremendous influence on learning.
- The *hippocampus* plays a significant role in information transfer to long-term memory.
- The *cingulate gyrus* serves as a message transfer channel to and from the limbic system.
- The *fornix* connects the hippocampus to the hypothalamus.

---

confusion among learners. Regardless, for the purpose of this book, what is most important is the function and role as opposed to the term used for the anatomical location.

Neurons

At the cellular level, neurons are built for efficiency in transmitting information. Neurons have three functional characteristics: (1) generate nerve impulses, (2) transmit nerve impulse to other parts of the cell, and (3) transmit signals to other cells and organs to create an effect. Neurons direct signals from cell to cell through dendrites and axons. Axons of one cell extend to the dendrites of the

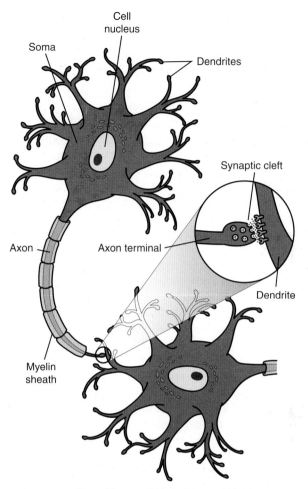

Fig. 5.5 Structure of a neuron. (From Heuston DH, Parkinson JW, Waterford Institute. *The Third Source: A Message of Hope for Education.* Salt Lake City, UT: Waterford Institute; 2011:235.)

next cell (Fig. 5.5). The dendrites are cell extensions that collect information from other cells. Neurons produce four types of signals for communication: input, trigger, conducting, and output. *Input signals* allows for the collection of messages; *trigger signals* integrate messages received; *conducting signals* send information to synapses; and *output signals* (commonly known as neurotransmitters) pass the information to the next neuron (Kolb and Whishaw, 2021). The signals from neurons are sent back and forth from cell to cell across the synapse, the gap between axons and dendrites. The process is enhanced by the myelin sheath—a coating over the axon and the neurotransmitters. The human brain has more than 100 billion neurons, with as many as 10,000 connections per neuron! Connections become a very important point in the next section when considering the brain structures related to learning.

BRAIN STRUCTURES AND LEARNING

Obviously, the brain is far more complex in its function and structure than the preceding discussion would suggest. However, this simplified approach (sensing, integrating, and responding) provides a useful framework for understanding the science of learning because the same process supports learning. The primary activity of human learning involves taking data in, integrating the data for meaning, and responding. These functions occur through trillions of data signals and networks between the neurons within the cerebral cortex. Various areas of the cerebral cortex play specific roles in the process of sensing, integrating, and responding as it relates to learning.

The function of sensing involves receiving auditory, visual, olfactory, and tactile data signals. The thalamus, located at the base of the cerebrum (see Fig. 5.4), serves as the brain's primary dispatch center for sensory data. It sends data signals (which are essentially nothing more than isolated bits of data) to the temporal and frontal regions of the cerebral cortex for integration.

The integrative process involves merging these data into clusters that become meaningful, such as visual recognition, language, sound, and images. These meanings are further integrated in various ways that become thoughts, ideas, and plans for action (Kolb and Whishaw, 2021; Zull, 2002). Considering the physiological function of various areas of the cerebrum, this process makes a great deal of sense. The frontal lobe is responsible for memory retention, higher level cognitive function, expressive speech, and voluntary eye and motor movement, while the temporal lobe controls receptive speech and the integration of visual, somatic, and auditory data. Interpretation of spatial data information occurs within the sensory cortex of the parietal lobe, while the processing of visual data occurs in the occipital lobe. The cerebellum also has a role in motor learning. Specifically, it has a role in timing and accuracy of movement, and it also participates in coupling of movements allowing for a smooth execution of multiple movements (Kolb and Whishaw, 2021); this coordination plays a significant role in the learning of psychomotor skills. As an example, learning to insert an intravenous catheter, requires the execution of several fine motor movements. The first few attempts are often awkward and clumsy, but with practice and repetition, the cerebellum facilitates the accuracy and smoothness of execution.

Responding refers to carrying out the action plans formed in the integration phase. Located centrally within the cerebrum are the paired basal ganglia, which are responsible for the initiation, execution, and completion of voluntary and automatic movement. These movements are necessary for a variety of actions including blinking, swallowing, running, and scratching, to name a few. Specifically related to learning, action movements are needed for the formation of speech and the ability to write, draw, and perform other related movements. The transfer of data signals (sensory input, integration, and motor response) is continuous and cyclic; sensory input triggers integrative activity, which triggers motor activity. The motor activity, in turn, serves as sensory data that start the cycle again. This cycle is automatic, and to a large extent it is subconscious. Fig. 5.6 shows the pattern and flow of sensory input, data integration, and motor response across the brain.

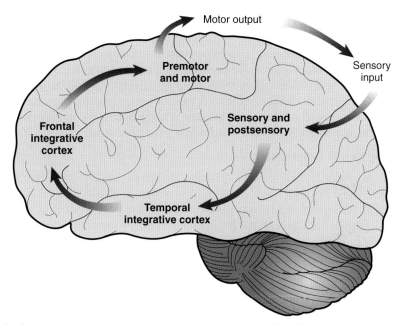

Fig. 5.6 Sensory input, data integration, and motor response. (Modified from Zull JE. *The Art of Changing the Brain: Enriching the Practice of Teaching by Exploring the Biology of Learning.* Sterling, VA: Stylus Publishing, LLC; 2002.)

THE LEARNING BRAIN

Sensing, Integrating, and Responding

Learning involves a combination of taking in new information and active thinking to translate the new information into meaning and appropriate actions. The three elements of sensing, integrating, and responding once again apply to this discussion.

In a learning situation, new information presents as auditory, visual, olfactory, and tactile data signals. The intake of information from the sensing brain has limited benefit or use unless the information is applied. In other words, there must be a process whereby the student not only receives knowledge, but also uses the knowledge in a way that requires the brain to actively integrate the information and transform it into understanding and meaning. Little is gained in situations where there is an intake of new information without using that information to stimulate thinking, create ideas, or generate an action plan. Likewise, the failure to intake information within the environment can occur due to a lack of attention or distraction. This can be useful during the learning process; with an active attention to material being learned, it is possible for the brain to ignore other data signals (such as hearing, but not attending to the sound of a lawnmower outside or ignoring background noise coming from another room).

Based on the preceding discussion, it should be obvious that integration of information is a necessary step for learning to take place. Two areas of the brain are involved with integration: the temporal integrative cortex and the frontal integrative cortex. The temporal integrative cortex involves memory of places and stories and information as facts. When new information comes in, the learner builds on existing knowledge—through existing neuronal networks. The frontal integrative cortex involves active mental energy, decisions, choice, and creativity. For this reason, learning is enhanced when there is balance between the two integrative sections. The outcome of a balanced approach is the transformation of a learner from a receiver of information to a producer of ideas (Zull, 2002).

Extending Neural Connections

The term *neuroplasticity* is used to describe the brain's ability to reorganize and restructure itself through the formation of new neural connections as a result of experiences (Dragansk and Gaser, 2004). In fact, the pattern of functional and structural connections within the brain changes in response to new experiences and learning; brain imaging during memory task performance illustrates this point (Popova et al., 2018).

Multiple variables influence neuroplasticity. Structural reorganization of the neurons results from increased protein synthesis. Also, repeated firing of a neuron's synapse leads to greater strength and efficiency in response as well as structural changes to the neuron; the changes include an increased density and length of the dendrite of the postsynaptic neuron (Kolb and Whishaw, 2021).

Another property of neurons is that they communicate with each other. When individual cells are activated at the same time, they establish connecting synapses or they strengthen existing ones. Thus, families of neurons form what is referred to as "cell assemblies" to represent units of behavior, and multiple cell assemblies link together ideas, allowing for a stream of thought. Repeated stimulation reinforces the activity of millions of synapses within cell assemblies and creates new ones—hence supporting the notion that brain plasticity represents change. Short-term memories to be converted into long-term memory neurons in the hippocampus are stimulated repeatedly (Collins, 2007). Interestingly, many brain changes occur as expertise is gained, including greater cognitive processing efficiency (compared to a novice), the use of different regions of the brain when solving problems, and greater efficiency in pattern recognition, allowing for rapid to immediate problem solving (Hill and Schneider, 2006). This partly explains the relative ease by which an expert provides complex clinical care compared to a novice.

Thus, neuroplasticity is an outcome of effective learning. When the brain is challenged with new information and problem solving, the integrative process of the mind involves clustering of data. In other words, the brain looks for patterns for meaningful organization and categorization of the information. New knowledge and information are matched to memory, extending and strengthening neural networks. This process facilitates the construction and extension of neuron connections; new knowledge structures are built with a new baseline for incoming information.

Seeking patterns represents an important underlying process associated with brain efficiency. The brain seeks patterns based on previous learning and experiences, allowing for very efficient responses to acquired knowledge and for efficiency in extending knowledge with new information. The pattern recognition can involve any of the senses; experts have greater efficiency in pattern recognition compared to novices, which allows for very fast or nearly automatic problem solving (Hill and Schneider, 2006).

However, sometimes mistakes are made with initial interpretation, and further information may be needed for clarification. For example, if a person walking on a path through the woods encounters an object that is long and thin, the brain may initially interpret the object as a snake, resulting in a fear response, and perhaps jumping out of the way to avoid harm. On further evaluation, it is determined that the shape is just a stick. This response results from the brain misinterpreting the visual cue and forming an initial response based on previous experiences with snakes. Likewise, a person may initially misidentify a wild raspberry plant for poison ivy because the brain searches for patterns—in this case three-leaflet pattern and growth in a shady wooded area. It requires further inspection and additional knowledge (such as the presence of thorny stems) to make the distinction.

Similarly, mistakes can be made in the thinking and learning process when information is incorrectly interpreted; this is particularly true when the brain anticipates something else based on pre-established patterns. For example, a nursing student may fail to notice nuances in drug administration information, particularly if he or she lacks awareness of such differences. Thus, the brain may incorrectly interpret new information based on preformed patterns. This is especially problematic if the student has built patterns on inaccurate or incomplete information. As an example, a student may believe that poor health outcomes among underrepresented minorities is based on genetic differences or their failure to take advantage of health services available to them. This information base must be clarified in order for the student to develop an accurate conceptual understanding of health disparities.

Variables Influencing Learning

As the previous section has demonstrated, learning is a very complex process. Not surprising, a number of physiological variables affect the learning process.

EMOTION

Earlier in this chapter, education neuroscience was introduced and described as an interrelationship between neuroscience, teaching, and psychological influences of the learner. Emotion represents a key psychological influence on the learner because of the effect on cognitive processing. Such effects include attention, perception, motivation, reasoning, and problem solving; these factors, in turn, affect learning and memory. Several neuroimaging techniques (such as functional magnetic resonance imaging, position emission tomography, electroencephalography, and functional near-infrared spectroscopy) have been used in neuroscience studies investigating the impact of emotion on learning (Tyng et al., 2017).

It has been noted several times throughout this chapter that sensing is one of the primary functions of the brain, and this involves the input of information. The emotional state of the learner influences the way sensory data are filtered in the brain. A positive emotional state favors conduction through the amygdala (see Fig. 5.4 and Box 5.1) and, as a result, information reaches the integrative areas of the brain. Positive states also enhance memory retention, particularly when there is something novel about the learning activity. In times of stress, fear, or anger, sensory data are largely sent to the lower-level reactive brain and data are not available for higher cognitive processing (Willis, 2010). This mechanism explains why it is very difficult to focus and learn in times of extreme stress and why individuals are more likely to be productive and learn when they are in a positive emotional state. The amygdala also has a powerful effect in committing emotionally charged events (both positive and negative) to long-term memory. This phenomenon is easily understood by the relative ease it is to recall a very happy, sad, or scary event in your life. Details of such events are often easy to recall, even decades later. Some of these events are based on an individual personal experience, such as the vivid memories one may have retained surrounding the birth of a child or death of a parent. Vivid memories may also be formed based on events that collectively affect a large group of people, or even an entire population. As one example, many adults can recall where they were and what they were doing when the news was emerging surrounding the events of 9-11.

Strategies to support the emotional regulation of learners has been described by Kuypers (2021) in her framework outlined in the curriculum, *The Zones of Regulation*. The four zones range from the Blue, Green, Yellow, and Red Zones as shown in Table 5.2. The Green Zone represents a state where the learner has an optimal level of alertness for academic pursuits, is relaxed, focused, and open to learning. Peak learning occurs in the Green Zone because a positive and calm emotional state allows information to reach the integrative areas of the brain, optimizing thinking and memory retention. The Blue Zone represents a low state of alertness and is associated with feelings of sadness, depression, not feeling well, fatigue, sleepiness, or boredom. Learners in a Blue Zone are exposed to information, but because they are in a low state of alertness, the data signals may not effectively reach a high-level integration state. Learners may also

TABLE 5.2 ■ **Zones of Regulation and Learning**

Zone	Alertness and Emotional State	Effect on Learning
Blue Zone	Low state of alertness; sadness, boredom, sleepy.	Suboptimal learning
Green Zone	Calm, relaxed state.	Optimal learning
Yellow Zone	Heightened state of alertness; anxiety, stress, excessive happiness.	Suboptimal learning
Red Zone	Extreme state; anger, rage, terror, devastation.	Learning not possible

The Zones of Regulation® and Learning.

struggle to recall information. Individuals in a Blue state need to "recharge," and this partly explains the need for engaging educational approaches, and the need for periodic breaks during learning. Alternatively, the Yellow Zone represents a heightened state of alertness and emotions, commonly associated with feelings of anxiety, stress, nervousness, and frustration, as well as excitement. Although learning may occur when a person is in the Yellow Zone, it often is not optimal for academic performance. The Red Zone represents an extreme heightened state of alertness and extreme emotions, such as terror, anger, rage, elation, or devastation. Learning rarely occurs during a Red Zone state because data signals essentially are directed to the lower reactive brain as opposed to the integrative cortex for higher-level thinking.

MOTIVATION

It has been long known that a fundamental element to facilitate learning is learner motivation. Nearly 100 years ago, Whitehead asserted that "There can be no mental development without interest" (Bonney and Sternberg, 2017). In his critical thinking work two decades ago, Facione (2000) wrote "We are best at learning what we most need and want to know" (p. 79), and the development of deep learning and critical thinking tends to be highest among those intrinsically motivated (Bonney and Sternberg, 2017). Nurse educators can relate to this statement, through experiences working with nursing students. In general, nursing students are highly motivated learners because of the direct application of the program content to the role of the nurse. Although students may demonstrate intrinsic motivation for learning (meaning they are engaged for the sake of learning or enjoyment), extrinsic motivation drives learning for many nursing students, meaning they are driven by external factors such as grades or recognition (Nakayoshi et al., 2021).

DOPAMINE

Another key variable associated with learning is dopamine, a neurotransmitter that facilitates the transmission of signals between neurons in the brain. Dopamine produces pleasurable feelings, and the amount of dopamine released is influenced by emotional states. An increased release of dopamine is triggered with positive experiences, and a drop in dopamine release can occur with negative experiences (Willis, 2010). This is an important principle because of dopamine's influence on learning. Dopamine acts as a reward mechanism in the brain related to learning and enhances the brain's translation of the information to memory. The nucleus accumbens, a dopamine storage structure, has been shown to release more dopamine when learners get answers right (which in turn creates a pleasurable feeling). Likewise, less dopamine is released when learners make a mistake or get an answer wrong (Salamone and Correa, 2002). This reward occurs when the brain is challenged and successful, when thinking about new information and solving new problems. Individuals with mastery in basic math would not get rewarded with increased dopamine release for correctly solving simple mathematical questions (such as $3 \times 5 = x$, or $12 + 6 = x$) because arriving at these answers does not represent a challenge. An individual is also not rewarded with dopamine when he or she attempts to solve a challenging problem and gets the answer wrong or is unable to make substantive progress. When there is no reward, motivation is reduced. Gee (2007) describes the power of this effect in the context of computer games with multiple levels that are increasingly difficult. The dopamine-enhanced pleasure of successfully achieving a level motivates the player to go on to the next, more challenging level.

MISCONCEPTIONS AND CLARIFICATIONS

Misconception: Rote memorization has no benefit to students and should be discouraged.	*Clarification:* Rote memorization of factual knowledge actually provides some benefits, because base information is easily and efficiently retrieved by the brain. Gaining a deep understanding of concepts and the ability to make generalizations from this understanding is supported by accurate, factual information. Rote memorization of facts does not, in itself, lead to higher order thinking, but provides the foundation to do so. The goal is for *learning with understanding* as opposed to *remembering and repeating facts*.

EXERCISE

Another variable that impacts learning is movement and exercise. It has been known for years that the brain is more active when the body is active and less active when the body is stationary (Sosa, 2010). Body movement and exercise increase the flow of blood to the brain, thereby increasing the delivery of oxygen and glucose to neurons. The obvious and direct benefit to learning is improved alertness and attention. However, there are many other indirect, and thus less obvious benefits. Exercise reduces insulin resistance and stimulates the release of growth factors that directly affect neuron health and neuroplasticity, which facilitates cognitive processing. Regular aerobic exercise has been shown to increase brain mass and the size of the hippocampus—which has a role in the transfer of learned information to long-term memory. The release of endorphins associated with exercise has a positive effect on motivation and mood, which facilitates learning. Regular exercise is associated with better sleep—another factor that is associated with learning. The association between movement and exercise and cognitive function has been demonstrated across the lifespan (Ullmann et al., 2021; Wei et al., 2021). This benefit is especially important during childhood when the brain is characterized by high neuroplasticity (Wick et al., 2021).

NUTRITION AND HYDRATION

The linkage between proper nutrition, hydration, and peak learning has been well documented. Carbohydrates are the main source of fuel for the brain.

The importance of healthy carbohydrate choices is based on the evidence that wide fluctuations in sugar levels hamper effective neurotransmission. An intake of an excessive amount of simple sugar triggers insulin release, which can cause drowsiness. In contrast, complex carbohydrates are associated with a slower breakdown and absorption of sugar, providing a steady release of fuel. Fats and proteins are needed to enhance healthy neurons, which in turn impacts neurotransmission. Optimal neurotransmission within the brain requires adequate hydration. A reduced hydrated state can lead to poor concentration, emotional changes, and reduced cognitive abilities, all of which have a negative impact on the ability to learn.

SLEEP

The brain depends on adequate sleep for proper function, thus an association between sleep and learning has long been understood. Sleep is involved with memory consolidation and brain plasticity. The process of consolidation involves a reorganization of information into stable memories, whereas plasticity refers to changes that occur when preexisting knowledge is modified as a result learning of new information. The sleep-deprived brain negatively impacts learning because of a lack of focus and attention, and the reduced ability to take in (sense) data from learning situations. Furthermore, when a person is in a sleep-deprived state, neurons are unable to efficiently coordinate data impulses, leading to impaired cognitive capacity. Sleep deprivation also impacts the brain's ability to store information into memory and memory recall (Cousins et al., 2019). Committing something recently learned to memory requires sleep—or, put another way, sleeping well the night after learning new information or a new skill is important for memory and future performance (Sosa, 2010). Memory consolidation (i.e., stabilization of a memory) takes place during sleep through the strengthening of neural connections. More recently, researchers have found evidence of the role of the hippocampus in short-term memory. Specifically, sleep spindles, which serve as "markers" for the brain's gateway traffic, help to encode memories from the hippocampus to other areas of the brain, and, in fact, primes the hippocampus to learn new information when a person wakes up. This activity has also been found as a result of napping (Talan, 2021). Although this process is poorly understood, it is thought that this process is linked to sleep waves during different phases of the sleep cycle. Memory recall (i.e., the ability to access something previously stored into memory) is also negatively impacted with insufficient sleep. Several other negative impacts of sleep deprivation are reported in the literature, including mood. Specific to learning, sleep-deprived students tend to have lower grades and are more likely to be depressed compared with their peers who get adequate sleep (Wolfson and Carskadon, 1998).

Conceptual Learning in the Nursing Discipline

Throughout this chapter, the discussion has focused on the science of learning without specific reference to conceptual learning. The science of learning provides substantial evidence related to the benefits of conceptual learning; thus, it should be increasingly clear that the conceptual approach is an opportunity for nurse educators to adopt strategies that enhance student learning. Ideally, this approach benefits learners not only while they are enrolled in nursing programs but also gives them the skills to emerge as efficient life-long learners throughout their career.

The massive volume of new knowledge generated throughout our society has made it impossible for any education program in any discipline to "cover" all the information in an academic program. With a greater understanding of how the brain learns, nursing educators must emphasize *learning with understanding* as opposed to *remembering and repeating facts*. Adopting the conceptual approach transforms the nursing education environment from a passive, static state with limited emotion or engagement into a vibrant, active, and challenging state with enhanced learning as an outcome. Given the preceding discussion about learning science, the relevance of this approach should be clear.

But what exactly is conceptual learning? Timpson and Bendel-Simso (1996) described conceptual learning as a process by which students learn to organize information into logical mental structures and become increasingly skilled at thinking. Fletcher and colleagues conducted a concept analysis of conceptual learning, representing an important contribution to the nursing literature. Based on this work the following definition is proposed:

Conceptual learning is a process in which learners organize concept-relevant knowledge, skills, and attitudes to form logical cognitive connections resulting in assimilation, storage, retrieval, and transfer of concepts to applicable situations, familiar and unfamiliar.

FLETCHER ET AL. (2019, p. 9)

The authors also identified five defining attributes of conceptual learning, including:

- Recognizing patterns in information
- Forming linkages with a concept
- Acquiring deeper understanding of a concept
- Discovering personal relevance and construction of value to self
- Aligning concepts to other situations

Conceptual learning requires the application of concepts and conceptual understanding to a situation, but this must be supported by a foundation of factual information. Thus, a hallmark of conceptual learning is that it necessitates the use of facts as opposed to a focus on facts, and the use of facts should be within the application of information in a larger context. Put another way, a deep understanding of concepts and the ability to make generalizations from those concepts is supported by facts and factual learning (Erikson and Lanning, 2014). It is the interaction of facts and concepts, within the context of clinical situations, that leads to deep understanding and the ability to transfer that information to other situations. Conceptual learning facilitates the formation of knowledge structures through neural connections and establishes patterns and connections in the brain. Over time, the conceptual learner develops an increased ability to translate previously learned information across multiple situations and contexts, and also develops the ability to take in new information and make connections between similar ideas and situations. In nursing, learning experiences should ideally be placed within the context of a clinical situation and be purposeful—in other words, learners should clearly recognize the benefit of what they are learning and how it applies to the practice of nursing. The work of Benner and colleagues (2010) confirmed the need for the contextualization for learning, as opposed to only learning facts. Placing the information to be learned in a clinical context, where students will actually see and apply the information, is necessary to optimize learning. Students must be exposed to clinical problems, and effective conceptual learning requires an investigative approach whereby they are challenged to think through multiple variables and to make important associations.

CONCEPTUAL THINKING AND EXPERT THINKING

The brain's ability to build a network of new neural connections during the learning process was discussed earlier in the chapter. The conceptual approach cultivates this process because the learner is making connections by actively thinking about the interrelationships of information to concepts and the interface of concepts across multiple situations and contexts. Patricia Benner's classic work *From Novice to Expert* (Benner, 1984) presented narratives describing thinking approaches among nurses across a spectrum of five stages of expertise: novice, advanced beginner, competent, proficient, and expert. Expert nurses, using their enormous background of experiences, have an accurate and intuitive grasp of situations and know how to respond, even in unique situations not previously encountered. This ability comes from well-honed cognitive skills—that is, the ability to focus on important data and recognize situations, synthesizing and analyzing the meaning of those data, and connecting this information to previous knowledge and experiences for an appropriate and seamless response. Bransford et al. (2000) point out that only a subset of one's total knowledge applies to any particular problem. Experts possess a rich and large reservoir of knowledge connected and organized around important concepts. They also have the skill to retrieve the applicable and appropriate knowledge related to a presenting problem, which is referred to as *conditionalized knowledge*. A key element of conceptual learning is honing the skill of conditionalized knowledge retrieval for problem solving.

Novices, by comparison, tend to have knowledge arranged in a list-like, disconnected fashion. They are unable to respond to complex problems effortlessly and accurately because they lack contextual experience, are more likely to have rigid or rule-based understanding of information, and tend to approach problem solving from a linear-thinking approach. Linear thinking is perpetuated when faculty approach teaching in a linear fashion (discussed in Chapter 6). New graduates who lack conceptual thinking skills are challenged during the transition to practice because they lack not only depth in clinical experiences but also the cognitive skills needed to make conceptual connections.

CONCEPTUAL LEARNING AND MEANINGFUL PATTERNS

A discussion regarding seeking patterns as a process associated with brain efficiency was presented earlier in this chapter. Conceptual organization allows an expert to see patterns and relationships not apparent to novice learners. Conceptual learning fosters the development of cognitive organization that is ultimately useful in specific situations in which the information is applicable, thus supporting deep understanding. The organization of information into a conceptual framework allows for an enhanced ability to transfer and apply information to a new situation (Fig. 5.7). The ability of the brain to transfer and apply information is hampered when knowledge lacks organization and presents as a set of disconnected facts. For this reason, a conceptual organization of information is foundational to clinical reasoning. The formation of clinical judgment and clinical reasoning in nursing requires an ability to make cognitive connections to past experiences and to learn from new experiences, thus building the neural connections related to nursing expertise. Clinical judgment represents a desired outcome of conceptual learning because of the trajectory from learning facts to thinking about concepts and the ability to make generalizations and linkages to principles. Tanner's Model of Clinical Judgment (Tanner, 2006) presents this process as occurring from the perspective of noticing, interpreting, responding, and reflecting within the situational context. The recognition of patterns related to specific conditions and situations is central to noticing and interpreting. This also closely links to the previous sections describing data intake and integrative processes within the brain. Responding represents the decision making and response that occurs in the brain. Reflecting, especially within the context of learning, represents the process of neuroplasticity (i.e., the formation of new neural connections within the brain as a result of experiences). Reflecting on these experiences drives deeper understanding for future learning.

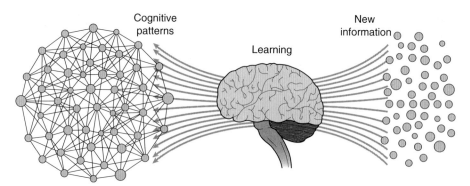

Fig. 5.7 Conceptual learning is characterized by patterns and multiple linkages. (Based on "Knowledge Information," Idiagram, © Marshall Clemens. Available at: http://www.idiagram. com/ideas/knowledge_integration.html.)

CONCEPTUAL APPROACH AND DEEP LEARNING

Conceptual learning encourages students to focus on big ideas (or concepts) and apply information or knowledge to specific situations. Learning complex subject matter, such as nursing and health care, requires the ability to transfer what has been previously learned into problem solving activities in the context of clinical situations. It does little good for students to learn about concepts in the absence of clinical examples, exemplars, or clinical application. Benner and colleagues (2010) frame this from the position of integrative teaching practices—in other words, framing student learning of concepts and exemplars in the context of a patient situation or clinical problem. Conceptual learning, particularly when framed in a clinical context, engages the learner with an application of information to things that are clearly relevant. This engagement and active application of information facilitates understanding and commits this understanding to long-term memory (Box 5.2).

What Does All of This Mean for the Nursing Faculty?

The preceding sections related to how the brain learns and conceptual learning underscore the need to rethink what is taught in nursing curricula and the best practices for teaching. Superficial coverage of large volumes of nursing content must be replaced with a deep understanding of concepts. However, there must be a sufficient number of clinical examples (exemplars) to allow in-depth study; this is necessary to allow students to fully grasp the concept (Bransford et al., 2000). The use of relevant clinical exemplars is crucial for gaining a conceptual understanding. That said, faculty should frame the exemplar learning through the conceptual lens as opposed to learning about an exemplar with the concept as an after-thought. As an example, the exemplar heart failure should be taught through the lens of the concept of perfusion as opposed putting heart failure in the "center ring" with perfusion as the side show. Over time, the use of concepts

---

BOX 5.2 ▪ Exemplar: Conceptual Learning in Action

Reyna, a nursing student, is learning about the concept of inflammation. Prior to the class, she read a chapter on the topic. In class she listened to a 15-minute presentation by the instructor and then viewed a 5-minute video highlighting the physiological response to inflammation. In her collaborative learning group, she shared a story about a time she experienced an inflammatory reaction and how her situation linked to what she had just learned. Her group then completed a case study featuring a situation involving a patient with an inflammatory condition and reinforced risk factors, typical presentation, and collaborative interventions for the situation. The instructor led a discussion session about the case, posing specific questions to the learning groups, including the interrelationship of the concept of inflammation to other concepts. The class concluded with a short reflective writing activity in which Reyna wrote about what she had learned about her new understanding of the concept.

to frame exemplars deepens conceptual understandings, thus making the case for an established set of concepts to be used over a curriculum.

TEACH WITH BALANCE

Traditionally, teaching has focused on delivering information in a student-passive approach. Assuming the students are paying attention, information is sent to the back portion of the cortex. The student must have an opportunity to integrate that information (using the frontal integrative cortex) to gain a deep and enduring understanding (Zull, 2002). Passive learning focusing on the memorization of facts is hard work because such an activity lacks context and associations. It is just as problematic when students are exposed to learning activities without an infusion of information. Conceptual learning should be balanced with a focus on the concept. A combination of concrete experiences involving reflection and student-centered learning where students are involved in abstract thought, problem solving, asking questions (thinking), hands-on activities, and activities requiring students to test their assumptions are central to conceptual learning. The application of such cognitive skills leads to more effective learning.

MISCONCEPTIONS AND CLARIFICATIONS

Misconception: A student-centered learning activity is essentially the same as conceptual learning.

Clarification: Conceptual learning is enhanced with student-centered activities, but conceptual learning does not automatically occur simply by designing a student-centered learning activity. Optimal conceptual learning occurs when:

- Learners build upon previous knowledge.
- The learning activity focuses on a concept and is tied to the clinical context.
- Students are fully engaged in the activity and perceive the learning activity as useful.
- Reflection is used to facilitate deep connections.
- The learning environment is safe.

PURPOSEFUL LEARNING

Conceptual learning must have a purpose that is apparent to the learner. Students' perception of the value of what is being learned influences motivation, which in turn influences what and how they learn (Ambrose et al., 2010). Transferring previous knowledge to a new learning situation is enhanced by not only creating a situation where students see the value or direct relationship to their area of study and the implications of why it is important, but that they can see the benefit while they are learning.

BUILD ON EXISTING KNOWLEDGE

Enhanced learning occurs when students can build on existing knowledge and apply new knowledge in purposeful ways. That the brain constructs new knowledge and understanding based on what a person already knows is an important principle that serves as a starting point for conceptual learning. It is also just as important for students to retrieve the necessary and appropriate knowledge to solve a problem. Preexisting knowledge should be considered an important starting point when creating conceptual learning activities. However, some learners have incomplete or inaccurate understandings, and this can interfere with new learning (Ambrose et al., 2010). For this reason, learning must be extended from a body of accurate information, thus, underscoring the importance of assessing students' baseline understanding.

REFLECTION

Reflecting on learning situations and experiences is one of the most important aspects of the conceptual approach and is a key to optimal learning in general. Reflection is a time to think about what has just happened in the learning situation and to actively contemplate things such as what was successful and what was not successful, how the situation differed from a previous situation, or how what was learned links to previously learned concepts. Reflective practice is a core component of the development of clinical judgment and clinical expertise (Tanner, 2006; Wright and Scardaville, 2021), thus students should be regularly encouraged to practice this. Further, faculty should build in reflection as part of conceptual teaching—including simulation—to optimize cognitive connections to concepts and clinical contexts.

MANAGE THE LEARNING ENVIRONMENT

Conceptual learning requires deep and purposeful thinking, and thus the learning environment must be free from unnecessary distractions and stress. Faculty must consider the tone of the classroom and the emotional state of students, as previously discussed. For example, it is not uncommon for first-semester nursing students to feel completely overwhelmed with the nursing school experience. Added to that may be feelings of inadequacy in a highly competitive cohort, along with personal stressors. Collectively these things matter and can impair learning. Elimination of unnecessary emotional stressors in the classroom or curriculum and creating an emotionally secure environment (one where learners feel respected by their teachers and free from potentially embarrassing situations) help to moderate other stressors.

EMOTION MATTERS

As in any learning situation, conceptual learning is optimized when learners are engaged and in a positive emotional state. Students do not typically become engaged when sitting and listening to a lecture. Therefore, nursing faculty are encouraged to teach using a variety of conceptual strategies that enhance learner engagement in pleasurable ways. The real trick is learning to foster an emotional connection to the material as opposed to just making learning fun. Novel teaching strategies that enhance curiosity are effective, as long as there is actual learning involved. Concepts taught using unfolding case studies (featuring characters familiar to the students) enhance a positive emotional connection to learning (Shuster et al., 2011), as does the incorporation of standardized patients, storytelling, and role-playing.

Summary

Educational neuroscience refers to the science of learning and includes the interrelationship between neuroscience, teaching practices, and psychology. The brain processes associated with learning include sensing, integrating, and responding. The brain's ability to learn is impacted by multiple factors such as emotion, dopamine, sleep, nutrition, and movement. Best practices in education have shown that learning is most effective when students link to and apply previous knowledge to new situations. Conceptual learning directly applies such principles; students learn concepts as big ideas and apply these to multiple increasingly complex situations and contexts, resulting in neuroplasticity. Faculty can enhance conceptual learning by teaching with balance, managing the learning environment, creating emotionally engaging learning activities that are purposeful, and promoting focused reflection.

References

Ambrose SA, Bridges MW, Dipietro M, et al. *How Learning Works. Research-Based Principles for Smart Teaching.* San Francisco, CA: Jossey-Bass; 2010.

Benner PB. *From Novice to Expert.* Addison Wesley: Menlo Park, CA; 1984.

Benner PB, Sutphen M, Leonard V, et al. *Educating Nurses: A Call for Radical Transformation.* San Francisco, CA: Jossey-Bass; 2010.

Bonney CR, Sternberg R. Learning to think critically. In: Mayer R, Alexander P, eds. *Handbook of Research on Learning and Instruction.* 2nd ed. New York, NY: Routledge; 2017.

Bransford JD, Brown AL, Cocking RR. *How People Learn: Brain, Mind, Experience, and School.* Washington, DC: National Academy Press; 2000.

Collins J. The neuroscience of learning. *J Neurosci Nurs.* 2007;39(5):305–309.

Connell JD. The global aspects of brain-based learning. *Educ Horiz.* 2009;88:28–39.

Cousins JN, Wong KF, Chee MWL. Multi-night sleep restriction impairs long-term retention of factual knowledge in adolescents. *J Adolesc Health.* 2019;65(4):549–557.

Dragansk D, Gaser C. Neuroplasticity: changes in grey matter induced by training. *Nature.* 2004;427 (22):311–312.

Erikson HL, Lanning LA. *Transitioning to a Concept-Based Curriculum and Instruction.* Thousand Oaks, CA: Corwin Press; 2014.

Facione PA. The disposition toward critical thinking: its character, measurement, and relationships to critical thinking skill. *Informal Log.* 2000;20:61–84.

Fletcher KA, Hicks VL, Johnson RH, et al. A concept analysis of conceptual learning: a guide for educators. *J Nurs Educ.* 2019;58(1):7–15. https://doi.org/10.3928/01484834-20190103-03.

Gee JP. *What Video Games Have to Teach Is About Learning and Literacy.* New York, NY: Palgrave Macmillan; 2007.

Hill NM, Schneider W. Brain changes in the development of expertise: neuroanatomical and neurophysiological evidence about skill-based adaptations. In: Ericsson KA, Charness N, Feltovich P,

Hoffman RR, eds. *The Cambridge Handbook of Expertise and Expert Performance.* New York, NY: Cambridge University Press; 2006:653–682.

Jensen E. *Brain-Based Learning: The New Paradigm of Teaching.* 2nd ed. Thousand Oaks, CA: Corwin Press; 2008.

Kolb B, Whishaw IQ. *Fundamentals of Human Neuropsychology.* 8th ed. New York, NY: Worth Publishers; 2021.

Kuypers L. *The Zones of Regulation*; 2021. http://www.zonesofregulation.com/index.html.

Nakayoshi Y, Takase M, Nitani M, et al. Exploring factors that motivate nursing students to engage in skills practice in a laboratory setting: a descriptive qualitative design. *Int J Nurs Sci.* 2021;8 (1):79–86.

Popova F, Kovacheva A, Garov P, et al. Adult brain activation during visual learning and memory tasks. An experimental approach to translational neuroscience. *J Eval Clin Pract.* 2018;24 (4):864–868.

Salamone JD, Correa M. Motivational views of reinforcement: implications for understanding the behavior functions of nucleus accumbens dopamine. *Behav Brain Res.* 2002;137:3–25.

Shuster G, Giddens J, Roerigh N. Emotional connection and integration: dominant themes among undergraduate nursing students using a virtual community. *J Nurs Educ.* 2011;50:222–225.

Sosa D. How science met pedagogy. In: Sosa D, ed. *Mind, Brain, and Education.* Bloomington, IL: Solution Tree Press; 2010.

Talan JB. A biological explanation for how napping enhances learning and memory. *Neurol Today.* 2021;21(6):1–30.

Tanner CA. Thinking like a nurse: a research-based model of clinical judgment in nursing. *J Nurs Educ.* 2006;45(6):204–211.

Timpson WM, Bendel-Simso P. *Concepts and Choices: Meeting the Challenges in Higher Education.* Madison, WI: Magna Publications; 1996.

Tyng CM, Amin HU, Saad M, et al. The influences of emotion on learning and memory. *Front Psychol.* 2017;8:1454.

Ullmann G, Li Y, Ray M, et al. Study protocol of a randomized intervention study to explore the effects of a pure physical training and mind-body exercise on cognitive executive function in independent living adults aged 65–85. *Aging Clin Exp Res.* 2021;33(5):1259–1266.

Wei J, Hou R, Xie L, et al. Sleep, sedentary activity, physical activity, and cognitive function among older adults: the National Health and Nutrition Examination Survey, 2011–2014. *J Sci Med Sport.* 2021;24(2):189–194.

Wick K, Kriemler S, Granacher U. Effects of a strength-dominated exercise program on physical fitness and cognitive performance in preschool children. *J Strength Cond Res.* 2021;35(4):983–990.

Willis J. The current impact of neuroscience on teaching and learning. In: Sosa D, ed. *Mind, Brain, and Education.* Bloomington, IL: Solution Tree Press; 2010.

Wolfson A, Carskadon M. Sleep schedules and daytime functioning in adolescents. *Child Dev.* 1998;69:875–887.

Wright J, Scardaville D. A nursing residency program: a window into clinical judgement and clinical decision making. *Nurse Educ Pract.* 2021;10. https://doi.org/10.1016/j.nepr.2020.102931.

Zull JE. *The Art of the Changing Brain.* Stylus: Sterling, VA; 2002.

CHAPTER 6

Concept-Based Instruction for the Classroom

Many aspects of the conceptual approach within nursing education are discussed in this book, including concepts, exemplars, a concept-based curriculum, conceptual learning, conceptual instruction, and assessment of learning. Ultimately, the effectiveness of the conceptual approach relies on faculty who provide an optimal platform for students to gain conceptual understandings, advanced thinking, and competency attainment. Successful implementation of the conceptual approach requires faculty to develop skills in concept-based teaching; this becomes the primary focus for faculty as the curriculum is implemented. The interrelationship between concept-based teaching and conceptual learning cannot be understated and must be fully understood. Effective concept-based instruction requires the instructor to understand:

- the **WHY** (why a conceptual teaching approach is needed);
- the **WHAT** (what are the key principles for conceptual teaching); and
- the **HOW** (how to plan, develop, and deliver concept-based instruction).

Faculty transitioning to concept-based teaching may feel anxious about the changes expected, a fact that has been well documented in the nursing literature (Repsha et al., 2020; Sportsman and Pleasant, 2017). However, good teaching is good teaching. Experienced faculty who are skilled teachers will find the transition relatively simple once an understanding of concept-based teaching is gained. This chapter provides an overview of concept-based teaching to support the conceptual approach and enhance student learning in the classroom setting. Additionally, specific examples of teaching strategies will help faculty grasp the ways content should be taught, ways to engage students with the content to be learned, and the role of the instructor to facilitate that learning.

Supporting Cognitive Frameworks

If you were to succinctly state the overarching goal of concept-based teaching ("why" we do it), it would be to *support the development of students' cognitive frameworks*. To elaborate further, the goals of concept-based teaching in the nursing discipline are for learners to (1) engage in conceptual learning, (2) develop higher order thinking skills, and (3) and apply their knowledge to other situations and contexts. These skills are needed to demonstrate competence in clinical practice.

Kavanagh and Sharpnack (2021) report a continued decline in the percentage of new graduates who demonstrated acceptable entry-level, initial competency—calling it a crisis in competency. Between 2016 and 2020 only 14% of new graduates demonstrated competence in a "safe" or "acceptable" range; between 2011 and 2015 the percentage in the acceptable range was 23% (Kavanagh and Szweda, 2017); this is compared to a 2005 report where 35% of new graduates were in an acceptable range (del Bueno, 2005). These findings support concerns that nursing education has not kept pace with the increasing complexity of health care and a very wide academic-to-practice gap. Although the conceptual approach does not represent a magic wand to address these concerns, it does represent a change in the direction needed for nursing education.

Concept-based teaching emphasizes the process of thinking which encourages students to recognize patterns and make connections to previously learned knowledge, leading to transferable understandings and the development of a robust cognitive framework. This is truly at the heart of conceptual learning. A detailed discussion on the neuroscience of learning and the relationship to conceptual learning was presented in Chapter 5; this information provides an important foundation on which faculty should begin their understanding of concept-based teaching. From a theoretical perspective, concept-based teaching aligns closely with constructivism, a learning theory in which cognitive frameworks are central to the learning process. New information is best understood when the learner can connect to their cognitive framework, which is based on previous knowledge and experiences. The existing knowledge held by the learner influences the way the learner makes sense of and interprets new information (Schunk, 2012). In other words, new information is incorporated into a learner's existing cognitive frameworks, leading to an expansion and refinement of the cognitive framework based on the new information.

Cognitive frameworks, also known as *mental frameworks* and *schemata*, help the learner organize and interpret information and integrate new information with previously learned knowledge (Deane and Asselin, 2015). This is part of the *integrating process* discussed in Chapter 5 through which learners sort and group data within their preexisting frameworks to make sense of, and to give meaning to, incoming data. As learners build their cognitive frameworks in nursing, the process of integrating incoming information into an existing schema from a nursing perspective becomes more efficient and accurate. Thus, what is taught and the teaching approaches used by faculty influence how students build cognitive frameworks in which to place and understand the information. Because a concept represents an overarching idea or principle, this approach aligns with the development and extension of students' cognitive frameworks by which students organize their thinking. This point becomes clearer when considering differences in cognitive frameworks in traditional and concept-based teaching approaches.

FACT-BASED, LINEAR TEACHING

A linear teaching approach places an emphasis on decontextualized content and facts. Content has been traditionally organized and taught using a linear

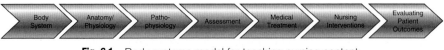

Fig. 6.1   Body systems model for teaching nursing content.

approach within many didactic nursing courses. For example, in an adult health nursing course, there is an emphasis on learning about health conditions, and nursing care for patients with such conditions. Content is typically framed around the health condition in a way similar to what is shown in Fig. 6.1. Anatomy, physiology, and pathophysiology are often presented as a basis to understand the health condition (and this may be repetitive information from other courses). Each condition has a list of risk factors, signs and symptoms, and laboratory/diagnostic studies included with a discussion on assessment. Medical treatment and nursing management are discussed, along with expected patient outcomes.

The presentation of information, especially when it lacks clinical context, results in students learning about nursing care as pieces of knowledge and information on the linear path and does little to provide relevance to the knowledge in practice situations. When content is organized and taught separately in a linear and decontextualized approach throughout the course and in other courses across the curriculum, students struggle to understand the significance and application of all the parts (Benner et al., 2010). Students tend to focus on the facts of information presented—and may perpetuate a surface approach to learning— described as "an extrinsic motivation to pass exams with the minimum effort" (Takase and Yoshida, 2021, p. 836). As a result of a linear, fact-based approach, many students build discrete cognitive patterns (similar to what is shown in Fig. 6.2) as opposed to the development of robust and complex cognitive frameworks. A systematic review evaluating learning approaches reported a significant negative correlation between surface approach learning and academic

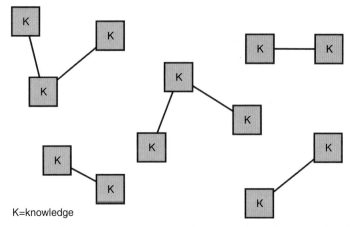

Fig. 6.2   Discrete cognitive linkages resulting from linear-based learning focused on knowledge.

achievement among undergraduate nursing students (Takase and Yoshida, 2021). Furthermore, with a linear approach faculty may miss opportunities to connect key content across the curriculum. As an example, safety, professionalism, and quality improvement are often taught in separate courses without consideration for how the content could be applied by students in meaningful ways within other courses.

CONCEPT-BASED TEACHING

In the conceptual approach, nursing content is organized and taught within a framework of concepts. As a result of concept-based instruction, students learn about the concept and then learn about exemplars with the concept serving as the overarching principle. Each exemplar is taught with an intentional link to the primary concept or concepts, allowing students to notice patterns and commonalities across like-conditions or clinical practice situations. In addition to focusing on the concept and exemplars, faculty guide students to make purposeful cognitive linkages to interrelated concepts across the curriculum. Furthermore, instruction is nested within a situational context—that is, within the practice of nursing. Effective conceptual teaching requires active thinking by the student which deepens and refines their understanding of the concept, leading to an expansion of their cognitive framework. Teaching with a conceptual framework helps students develop cognitive patterns that look similar to those demonstrated in Fig. 6.3—which is in stark contrast to the discrete cognitive patterns associated with the linear approach (see Fig. 6.2). The conceptual approach also aligns with a "deep learning approach" (described as students' intrinsic motivation for learning). Researchers report a significant positive correlation between deep approach learning and academic achievement among undergraduate nursing students (Takase and Yoshida, 2021).

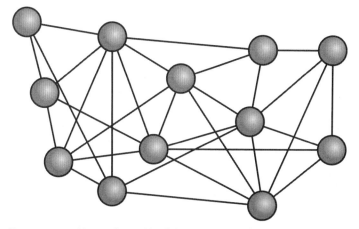

Fig. 6.3 Pattern recognition and cognitive linkages resulting from the conceptual approach.

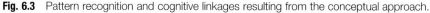

MISCONCEPTIONS AND CLARIFICATIONS

Misconception: An easy way to adapt a conceptual teaching approach is to use body systems as concepts, and then teach content around body systems.	**Clarification:** Renaming body systems as concepts does not result in conceptual teaching. Although some concepts relate to body systems other important concepts do not align with body systems. Concept-based teaching requires a specific and purposeful approach to facilitate thinking by linking concepts to supporting content and the formation of generalizations.

WHY ARE COGNITIVE FRAMEWORKS IMPORTANT?

Based on the previous sections, it should become obvious that a distinct difference between a traditional teaching approach and the conceptual approach is the development of a more comprehensive cognitive framework, leading to advanced thinking skills. These cognitive skills facilitate the transferability of information to other concepts and are a necessary component to make generalizations. According to Benner et al. (2009), the expert nurse has a deep understanding of the total situation and is able to focus immediately on salient aspects without wasting time and energy on a large range of alternative solutions.

Advanced thinking skills underlie the ability to make sound clinical judgments. The process of clinical judgment developed by Tanner (2006) was shown in Fig. 1.4 in Chapter 1. A nurse's response to a clinical situation is influenced by his or her knowledge, past experiences, and knowledge of the patient. This represents a baseline with regard to what the nurse expects to see and thus the ability to *notice* when patterns are inconsistent. Recognizing inconsistencies by applying a thorough understanding of each concept, the nurse gains additional information to correctly *interpret* the situation and *respond* appropriately. The actions taken during the respond step are dependent on the health care environment in which the nurse is working. The expert nurse then *reflects* on this experience, which further expands the nurse's knowledge and experience. The ability to make clinical judgments in this way is enhanced through conceptual thinking skills because of the cognitive connections students make when encountering new information. Reflective thinking, however, must be purposeful in this process for the base of knowledge and experience to grow (Tanner, 2006). Concept-based teaching strategies are designed to help students think intuitively on a higher level and to thus, support their evolving clinical judgment. Unfortunately, as noted before, most nursing graduates are not able to think at the levels required in the current health care environment (Kavanagh and Sharpnack, 2021).

An expectation to demonstrate thinking at a higher level is driving significant change by the National Council of State Boards of Nursing (NCSBN). The research-based, clinical judgment model in nursing (Dickison et al., 2016) is being used as a basis to develop and evaluate questions that measure clinical judgment as part of the Next Generation NCLEX Project (NCSBN, 2021). Ultimately this work will influence NCLEX-RN in the near future.

Key Principles for Conceptual Teaching

The previous section established why concept-based teaching is needed—that is, to support the development of cognitive frameworks among students. A strong foundation of knowledge for each of the concepts is needed to establish and develop the cognitive frameworks. This section discusses the "what"—*what are the key principles for conceptual teaching*? Faculty are often surprised to learn that much of the content taught in a traditional nursing curriculum is also taught in a concept-based curriculum. The distinct differences include the intentional framing of content within concepts, and the selective use of exemplars to deepen students' understanding of the concept. Concepts and exemplars are the focal points to organize instructional content. With this in mind, five general principles are associated with concept-based teaching and include:

1. Teach the concept using a concept presentation format.
2. Teach designated exemplars for each concept.
3. Integrate teaching within situational context.
4. Link new information to preexisting understandings.
5. Engage students.

MISCONCEPTIONS AND CLARIFICATIONS

Misconception: Once a concept-based curriculum is in place, all faculty will automatically teach the curriculum in the way it was intended.

Clarification: Many faculty are comfortable teaching in a traditional, linear manner and may not initially be open to learning new teaching methodologies. Intentional faculty development will be needed to enhance the skill and confidence among faculty members as part of a transition process.

THE CONCEPT PRESENTATION

In order for students to gain a foundational understanding of the concepts, a *concept presentation* must be intentionally incorporated into the curriculum. As part of curriculum planning, a determination is made regarding which course(s) the concept presentation will occur for each concept. The sequencing of concept presentations is highly variable, depending on the curriculum design. In some curriculum plans, all concept presentations may occur within the first semester; in other programs, the concept presentations may be spread out over multiple semesters.

Regardless of sequencing, a consistent approach should be used for the concept presentation across all courses to enhance the development of students' understanding and for the sake of curriculum integrity. A concept presentation includes many of the elements associated with a concept analysis, as described in

Chapter 3. Ideally, faculty will agree to use a standardized template to develop concept presentations; doing so helps to achieve consistency, which will accelerate student's grasping of concepts. Examples of templates that can be used to develop the concept presentations are presented in Tables 6.1 and 6.2.

Once faculty agree on a standardized outline or template to use for the concept presentation, a lesson plan is developed for each concept, incorporating a variety of teaching strategies. Learners benefit when a variety of teaching strategies are used. Developing a lesson plan for the concept presentation is helpful to create a balanced and purposeful learning experience for students. Table 6.3 shows an

TABLE 6.1 ■ Concept Presentation Template for Health and Illness Concepts

Topic	Description
Concept Definitions	A clear definition of the concept should be included so students (and faculty) are all working from a common definition; concept definitions can be easily found in the literature.
Scope or Categories of Concept	All concepts have scopes or categories; a scope is like a continuum (such as hyperthermia, normothermia, or hypothermia), whereas categories are discrete distinctions (such as types of infections).
Populations at Risk/ Individual Risk Factors	Students should gain an understanding of what populations or individuals are most likely to have or to develop a problem with the concept, which is a critical skill for *noticing* as it relates to clinical judgment; help students differentiate populations at risk as opposed to individual risk factors.
Physiologic Processes and Consequences	Normal physiologic processes and the physiologic basis for dysfunction and consequences (i.e., what the individual experiences).
Assessment • History • Examination findings • Diagnostic tests	At the concept level, this section helps the student identify the individual's status as it relates to the concept (optimal functioning or dysfunction); again, this understanding is critical for clinical judgment.
Clinical Management • Primary prevention • Screening • Collaborative interventions	Students must gain a clear understanding of what they should do when encountering the health care recipient as it relates to the concept, which is also a critical element of clinical judgment; this comprehensive look at preventative, screening, or treatment options is performed to enhance or maintain optimal function or treat in situations of dysfunction and is not focused at the disease level but rather at the concept level; when exemplars are taught, the elements within this section should easily connect.
Interrelated Concepts	Students should consider how the concept links to other concepts; many concepts are closely interrelated (e.g., perfusion and gas exchange); purposeful learning about these interrelationships establishes the cognitive patterns needed for making future connections.
Common Exemplars	Every concept has multiple exemplars although only a few are formally taught. Exemplars are taught by linking to the concept.

TABLE 6.2 ■ Concept Presentation Template for Professional Nursing and Health Care Concepts or Health Care Recipient Concepts

Topic	Description
Concept Definitions	A clear definition of the concept should be included so students (and faculty) are all working from a common definition; concept definitions can be easily found in the literature.
Scope or Categories of Concept	All concepts have scopes or categories; a scope is like a continuum (such as novice to expert); categories are discrete distinctions (such as leadership styles).
Attributes	Attributes are the critical elements used to correctly identify the concept; they are like the "rule" for acceptance; attributes are essential for clarification related to recognition of the concept in practice.
Theoretical Links	Many of the professional nursing concepts and patient attribute concepts have strong links to a theory or theories, such as Tanner's Model of clinical judgment; students should gain a perspective on these theories to better understand the concept.
Context to Nursing and Health Care	The context to nursing and health care should help the student gain an understanding of the situational context in which the concept will be seen and how it applies to the practice.
Interrelated Concepts	Students should consider how the concept links to other concepts; many concepts are closely interrelated (e.g., quality and safety), and purposeful learning about these interrelationships establishes the cognitive patterns needed for making future connections.
Common Exemplars	Every concept has multiple exemplars although only a few are formally taught. Exemplars are taught by linking to the concept.

TABLE 6.3 ■ Sample Lesson Plan for the Concept of Perfusion

Focus Area	Teaching Strategies/Activities	Learning Outcome
Concept Introduction	• Instructor: Introduce concept definitions, categories (e.g., central perfusion and local perfusion) and scope (e.g., no perfusion, reduced perfusion, and optimal perfusion). • Learning Groups: Students share what they have previously learned or seen that links to perfusion categories and/or scopes.	Clearly articulates the concept
Concept Identification	• Instructor: Present populations at highest risk for perfusion problems; clarify how these are similar and different from individual risk factors. • Learning Groups: Students complete a table identifying common individual risk factors across the life span; groups report and the instructor clarifies answers. • Instructor: Present a profile of four persons; students identify individual risk factors for each person.	Recognizes persons with optimal perfusion, those at risk, and those who are experiencing poor perfusion

Continued

TABLE 6.3 ■ Sample Lesson Plan for the Concept of Perfusion—cont'd

Focus Area	Teaching Strategies/Activities	Learning Outcome
	• Instructor: Presentation/review focused on how perfusion can become impaired and physiological consequences with impairment; shows a short video that clearly illustrates this process.	
	• Learning Groups: Students review assessment skills previously learned in their health assessment class and link data to central perfusion, local perfusion, or both.	
	• Instructor: Show photos depicting clinical findings of impaired perfusion; the students describe the relevance of the signs.	
	• Learning Groups: Students complete a worksheet on common diagnostic tests to evaluate perfusion (central and local).	
Clinical Management	• Learning Groups: Assign half the groups to locate recommended health promotion strategies from Healthy People 2030 (each group has a different age group) and half the groups to locate recommended screening guidelines from the USPSTF (each group has a different age group); the group's report.	Initiates appropriate interventions and assesses patient outcome
	• Instructor: Present lecture about clinical treatment guidelines for perfusion problems—procedures, surgical interventions, and pharmacotherapy.	
Transferable Ideas	• Learning Groups: Students will identify up to five curriculum concepts and draw a concept map showing interrelated connections.	Application of principles to other concepts and clinical conditions
	• Learning Groups: Students will brainstorm medical conditions they are aware of that represent perfusion problems and identify if it represents a central or peripheral perfusion problem; the instructor will clarify answers and add to lists generated for further consideration.	
Notes	• After the concept overview, the following exemplars will be used to deepen the students' understanding of perfusion:	
	• Heart failure,	
	• Acute myocardial infarction,	
	• Peripheral vascular disease.	

USPSTF, U.S. Preventive Services Task Force.

example of a lesson plan for a didactic classroom concept presentation for *Perfusion* and Table 6.4 shows an example of a lesson plan for a didactic classroom concept presentation for *Health Promotion*. Notice that the sample lesson plans represent a balance between faculty-led and student-centered activities. The plans incorporate a situational context for learning enhancement and purposeful

TABLE 6.4 ■ **Sample Lesson Plan for the Concept Health Promotion**

Focus Area	Teaching Strategies/Activities	Learning Outcome
Concept Introduction	• **Individually/Pairs/Groups:** Write out one or two sentences of what the terms health promotion, health, wellness, and disease mean to you. Share your definitions with the person sitting next to you. Combine your ideas. Now find another group of two. As a group of four, share your ideas about these terms. Review definitions. How do your ideas link to the definitions you found? • **Instructor:** Share the World Health Organization definitions with the class; how are their definitions similar?	Student clearly articulates the meaning of the concept and related terms.
Scope of Concept	• **Instructor:** Show visual depiction of Primary, Secondary, and Tertiary Prevention. In discussion format, ask student for examples and differentiation of each. • **Instructor:** Show a visual depiction of the trajectory of health promotion (individual, family, community, etc.) as well as life span of individuals. Lead discussion regarding health promotion on these trajectories, noting obvious differences and similarities.	Articulates the three primary categories and application among various individuals and groups.
Concept Attributes	• **Instructor:** Review four attributes of health assessment—optimizes health, evidence-based, patient/family/community orientation, culturally relevant. • **Learning Groups:** Students review a common health promotion initiative (such as smoking cessation or breastfeeding for infant health) and identify evidence of all attributes within the health initiative. • **Instructor:** Show slide of the WHO 12 Tips to Be Healthy and the 3 Pillars of Health Promotion. Discuss each of the slides in context of visibility within society, and challenges in implementation.	Recognizes consistent pillars and attributes present in all health assessment priorities.
Theoretical Links	• **Instructor:** Presents brief lecture on common health promotion models.	Attains a beginning-level awareness of how theory affects health promotion activities.

Continued

TABLE 6.4 ■ **Sample Lesson Plan for the Concept Health Promotion—cont'd**

Focus Area	Teaching Strategies/Activities	Learning Outcome
Nursing Role in Health Promotion	• **Instructor:** Lead discussion regarding differences in health promotion assessment between individual, family and community-based assessments. • **Learning Groups:** Students will complete jigsaw activity featuring the most common interventions to support health promotion and specific role of the nurse within these interventions.	Initiates appropriate interventions to achieve patient outcomes.
Transferable Ideas	• **Learning Groups:** Students will review an assigned health promotion policy. Using specific guidelines, they will determine how evidence, health disparities, patient education, and health care economics apply to the assigned health promotion policy answers and add to lists generated for further consideration	Application of principles to other concepts and clinical conditions
Notes	After the concept overview, the following exemplars will be used to deepen the students' understanding of health promotion: • Physical activity, • Smoking cessation, • Blood pressure screening.	

linkages to past learning that connects to the students' existing cognitive frameworks, which are critical elements to include in any lesson plan to enhance learning (Brown et al., 2014). Also note that the concept presentations do not include a presentation of exemplars, but students are encouraged to consider possible exemplars that link to the concept.

Intentional connections to other concepts should be included in the lesson plan as well. One could make the case that all concepts connect to each other in some way, so the focus should be on the concepts that have the closest connection and greatest impact on the primary concept being discussed. The discussions should focus on the commonly associated interrelated concepts that comprise the enduring understandings of a concept that may apply to most patients or clinical situations. Other interrelated concepts emerge when the concept is applied to a specific clinical context or specific patient situation.

TEACHING EXEMPLARS

After the concept presentation, exemplars are taught to give students an opportunity to understand the concept more deeply. An exemplar is a specific health condition or clinical situation in which the concept under study would be present. Referring to Fig. 6.4, there are multiple exemplars that represent the concept

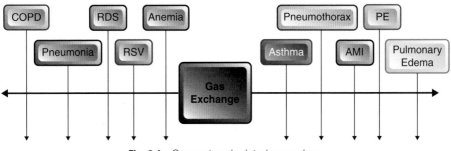

Fig. 6.4 Concept and related exemplars.

of gas exchange. Faculty should teach the designated exemplars that best represent the concept (according to the curriculum plan) and resist the temptation to teach all exemplars from a previous curriculum. Teaching an excessive number of exemplars results in content saturation, with faculty reverting back to intense lectures and students engaging in rote memorization. This outcome minimizes the benefits of the concept-based approach (Giddens and Brady, 2007). Students have many opportunities to learn additional exemplars and to make linkages to concepts during clinical experiences.

Exemplars are taught by intentionally linking the exemplar to the concept, other interrelated concepts, and to previous understandings. Like concepts, exemplars are taught using a variety of student-centered learning activities and framed within a clinical context. When presented in the context of a specific patient or practice situation, exemplars provide a deeper and more meaningful understanding of the concept, thereby enhancing students' skills in knowledge transferability.

INTEGRATE TEACHING IN SITUATIONAL CONTEXT

One of the traits of expert nursing faculty is integrated teaching—that is, framing what is being learned in a situational context (Benner et al., 2010). The importance of situational context has been mentioned in the two previous sections and in Chapter 5. Situational or contextual learning helps students understand how the information they are learning is applied in practice, such as with a unique patient or professional nursing situation. "Putting new knowledge into a *larger context* helps learning" (Brown et al., 2014, p. 6). Context enhances conceptual learning because it helps the learners gain an understanding of why the information is important and facilitates the learners' ability to transfer ideas from one situation to another. In other words, they can see the relevance of the information they are learning, which enhances learner interest and motivation. Situational learning can be successfully applied in classroom settings using a number of teaching strategies including case studies, virtual patients, and simulation, to name a few.

Box 6.1 illustrates how easily a classroom activity can be framed within a situational context. Compare the information shared in Box 6.1 to an

---

BOX 6.1 ■ Exemplar: Situational Context in Action

Jason, a nursing instructor, prepares a concept presentation for the concept of Gas Exchange. As part of the learning activity, he provides a clinical presentation of two people—an older adult and a young child—both of whom have impaired gas exchange. In small groups, students discuss the clinical presentation, offer their thoughts, and then decide which data (provided on a worksheet) could be attributed to impaired gas exchange. Students are encouraged to confirm their decisions with a textbook resource. Students then discuss the cause of the symptoms, from a physiological perspective, as well as how the symptoms are similar and different based on age. Jason tells the students that recognizing impaired gas exchange in people of all ages is an expected competency in clinical practice.

---

all-too-common teaching scenario where students are presented with a Power-Point slide presenting common clinical findings of impaired gas exchange in a bulleted list. Students write down the list of words (and/or demand the slides) so they can memorize the information for their upcoming test. In this case, the information is merely presented as a list of words and lacks clinical context. Such an approach does little to engage students or help them gain an understanding how the concept presents in a clinical situation.

LINK TO PREEXISTING UNDERSTANDING

As discussed at the beginning of the chapter, faculty can facilitate conceptual learning by providing opportunities for students to construct new knowledge from previous understanding. Thus, the fourth principle for concept-based teaching is intentional linkages to past learning and preexisting understandings as part of a lesson plan. It is important, however, that students are building on accurate pre-existing knowledge. Students may have inaccurate understandings for a number of reasons including misunderstandings with previous learning that was not corrected, changes in knowledge since the student initially learned something, or even misconceptions or inaccurate understandings based on deeply held perceptions and beliefs, even when presented with updated or alternative information. Prior knowledge based on a belief system can be difficult to unlearn (Hardin and Richardson, 2012). As an example, when learning about evidence and best practices for infant sleeping, a nursing student may hold a strong belief about infant co-sleeping based on his or her personal parenting experience. This experience influences the student's pre-existing knowledge.

Thus, it is sometimes useful to have a "refresher" of pre-existing understandings before or as part of the introduction of new information. This can be done in several ways including reading assignments, review worksheets, refresher quizzes, a short questionnaire administered at the beginning of the class (Hardin and Richardson, 2012), or classroom discussion. Faculty should resist the temptation, however, of reteaching previously learned content. Part of the role of the instructor is to clarify and redirect students with inaccurate understandings. As the student progresses through the nursing program, the meaning of any one concept will expand as it is applied to different populations and settings as well as to increasingly complex situations.

ENGAGE STUDENTS

The fifth principle for conceptual teaching is student engagement through student-centered learning. The term "student-centered learning" closely aligns with what is referred to as inquiry-based instruction in the education discipline literature. Constructivist learning theory supports the creation of meaning and development of cognitive knowledge structures based on experiences. Inquiry-based learning requires active participation by learners, thus providing the experiences needed for knowledge development (Loyens & Rikers, 2017). The instructor must abandon teaching practices that emphasize content and facts and adopt student-centered approaches that require active application or analysis of information, thus linking learning to concepts within the context of nursing practice. Learning activities should actively engage students, focus on a clinical situation, require students to think and be meaningful. Students should clearly understand how the activity contributes to their learning.

Student-centered learning is often done through cooperative learning activities. In cooperative learning, students are placed into small groups, and they work together on a specific problem or activity to learn the content. The specific learning method and size of groups can vary—ranging from formal to informal learning. Faculty are often reluctant to have students work in learning groups for fear students may not participate or lack the ability to complete the work correctly. However, hundreds of studies have been conducted related to cooperative learning, and the general findings demonstrate positive effects (Slavin, 2017). The power of collaborative learning is that students engage on a different level than they do when listening to a lecture. When students work in teams, the combined effect of different brains thinking together—particularly if they are encouraged to look for information online or in their textbook—typically results in accurate work. The role of the faculty member, as the facilitator of learning, is to provide guidance as students complete the activities and to redirect if students are arriving at incorrect conclusions.

Designing Concept-Based Learning Activities for the Classroom

Using the five principles of conceptual teaching, discussed in the preceding section, faculty can successfully develop concept-based learning activities (CBLAs) to support conceptual learning in the didactic (classroom or online) settings. This process starts by developing a lesson plan. Components of a lesson plan include learning outcomes, pre-class assignments, teaching/learning strategies, and evaluation of learning. Planning is needed to ensure that the instructional and learning strategies facilitate students' achievement of the desired outcomes. The development of CBLAs for clinical education is discussed in Chapter 7.

LEARNING OUTCOMES

Lesson planning for class sessions begins with the development of intended learning outcomes. Learning outcomes outline what students are expected to learn as a result of the course module, class session, a specific learning activity, or assignment. The outcomes should clearly align to the course learning outcomes and also typically refer to the specific concept, exemplar, and/or competency under study. As a reminder, program-level outcomes and course outcomes are written as part of curriculum development. Competencies are outcome statements associated with concepts and domains. This information is discussed in Chapter 4 and Fig. 4.2 illustrates the alignment of student learning outcomes from program to course, to specific class sessions and learning activities, with a specific linkage to concepts/domains, and competencies.

Three domains (or classifications) of learning outcomes known as Blooms's taxonomy have been historically used by educators to plan and evaluate learning and include the cognitive (thinking) domain, psychomotor (skill) domain, and the affective (beliefs/values) domain (Anderson and Krathwohl, 2001; Scheckel, 2016). These domains are hierarchical—in other words (less complex or less skill to greater complexity or skill) and should reflect the progressing expectations in knowledge and skill of learners as they progress through a program. Box 6.2 presents a description of these three domains and the hierarchical categories.

BOX 6.2 ■ Learning Outcome Domains and Hierarchical Categories

Creating	Naturalization	Internalization
↑	↑	↑
Evaluating	Articulation	Conceptualizing
↑	↑	↑
Applying	Precision	Valuing
↑	↑	↑
Understanding	Manipulation	Responding
↑	↑	↑
Remembering	Imitation	Receiving

Cognitive Domain:	**Psychomotor Domain:**	**Affective Domain:**
Learning outcomes that reflect thinking	Learning outcomes that reflect skill development	Description: Learning outcomes that reflect values, beliefs, and attitudes

SELECTING TEACHING AND LEARNING STRATEGIES

After developing learning outcomes for the module, class session, learning activity, or assignment, specific strategies are planned to ensure students achieve the desired outcome. Because of the wide range of learning preferences among learners, a variety of teaching and learning activities should be planned (as opposed to doing the same strategies over and over again). Pre-class assignments typically include a reading assignment or some other preparatory work. Many teaching strategies can be used to promote student-centered conceptual learning (Box 6.3); most of these strategies are also used in a traditional classroom. However, it is not the teaching strategy itself that makes it "concept-based" because a teaching strategy is a method, not the outcome. Conceptual teaching incorporates a number of teaching strategies focused on a concept—with an emphasis on conceptual understanding. Teaching strategies should help students construct a cognitive framework based on concepts, and thus concepts are the unifying, driving focus of the teaching techniques selected.

Short collaborative CBLAs integrated within faculty-led discussions (as shown in Tables 6.3 and 6.4) are very effective for various aspects of the concept or exemplar presentations. A description of several strategies that can be applied to various aspects of concept or exemplar learning as individual or collaborative learning activities are presented in the sections that follow.

Instruction Based on Inquiry

Inquiry-based instruction is a term that represents four classic instructional methods: inquiry-based learning, problem-based learning, project-based learning, and case-based learning. Common to all four methods, students learn principles and concepts by working through a project or case. The highly contextualized state of the problem, project, or case enhances learning further because it is realistic and meaningful; the instructor serves as a facilitator and learning coach (Loyens and Rikers, 2017).

Case-based learning is the most common of inquiry-based instructional methods used in the health professions—including nursing. Case studies

---

BOX 6.3 ■ Teaching Strategies That Support Conceptual Learning

■ Simulation	■ Audiovisual (videos, songs)
■ Traditional Case Study	■ Storytelling
■ Unfolding Case Study	■ Role Play
■ Virtual Communities	■ Concept Analysis
■ Gaming	■ Concept maps
■ Jigsaw	■ Case writing
■ Debate	■ Classroom response systems
■ Guided Questions	■ Pair and Share Discussions
■ Concept assessment	■ Compare and Contrast
■ Risk Factor Assessment	■ Vignettes

BOX 6.4 ■ Example of a Virtual Family

The Belmont Family

- Deborah, age 35 years, height 5'1", weight 175 lb, works full time as an auditor for the state, and volunteers for her children's activities.
- Alvin, age 38 years, height 5'9", weight 250 lb, works full time as a truck driver. Is out of town 3 days a week, smokes two packs of cigarettes a day, takes medication for depression and hypertension, recently diagnosed with diabetes mellitus type 2.
- Austin, age 7 years, Jennifer's son from a previous marriage; easygoing personality, active in sports, good student, has exercise-induced asthma for 3 years, frequent upper respiratory tract infections in the winter.
- Oliva, age 2 years, Jennifer and Alvin's daughter. Attends daycare, has frequent ear infections. Parents have difficulty controlling her temper tantrums.
- Frank, age 72 years, is Alvin's father and recently moved in with the family. Has mild dementia, frequent falls, osteoporosis, and severe emphysema (smoker for 60 years). Broke hip last year; currently uses a walker.

---

typically focus on a single situation relevant to the topic being studied, although an unfolding case study presents a situation over time. Another alternative is the use of "standardized virtual patients" which are fictional characters that support learning throughout a course or curriculum. Students become familiar with each standardized virtual patient (his or her health history, family situation, and living situation, for example), and faculty use these virtual patients on an ongoing basis for a number of learning activities. Several examples of the use of standardized virtual patients have been reported in the nursing literature (Croteau et al., 2011; Curran et al., 2009; Giddens, 2007; Walsh, 2011). Box 6.4 presents an example of basic biographical information for a standardized virtual family. A complete profile about the family and additional artifacts such as photos, videos, and other supporting information is developed and placed on an online platform.

Classroom Discussion

Classroom discussions can be a very useful way to engage students. There are a variety of approaches that can be effectively used for discussions such as large group discussions, small group discussions, discussions led by the instructor, peer-led discussions by the students themselves, structured discussions with guiding questions to facilitate discussion (often termed "quality talk"), and even approaches with less structure such as a book club discussion (Murph et al., 2017).

Guided questions can be used with any part of a concept presentation. This teaching strategy gives students the opportunity to actively engage in thinking about the concept and what it means to them. Guided questions encourage students to connect what they already know to the new information they are learning and provide faculty with valuable information about the students' current understanding of the topic. Box 6.5 presents an example of guided questions used in a concept introduction of Collaboration.

BOX 6.5 ▥ Guided Discussion Questions for the Concept of Collaboration

- Based on your readings and/or previous experiences, what does the word "collaborate" mean to you?
- Describe a situation in which you experienced effective or successful collaboration with others. Why was the collaboration effective or successful?
- Describe a situation in which you experienced ineffective or unsuccessful collaboration with others. Why was it unsuccessful?

BOX 6.6 ▥ Scope of the Concept Motivation

In your learning groups, share examples or situations in health care management you have seen or heard about that illustrate the concept of *Motivation* across the trajectory of no motivation to intrinsic motivation.
- Intrinsic Motivation
  Example/Situation:
- Extrinsic Motivation with self-determination
  Example/Situation:
- Extrinsic Motivation without self-determination
  Example/Situation:
- No Motivation
  Example/Situation:

Drawing on Past Experiences

All students have previous experiences or are aware of the experiences of others. Use past experiences to bridge students' thinking to new situations. Box 6.6 provides an example of a collaborative in-class learning activity that directs students to discuss the various dimensions of motivation in the context of health care management, based on past experiences they have seen or heard about. In this specific example, the learning activity helps students learn about the scope or categories of the concept, as part of the concept overview.

Risk Factor Assessment

Box 6.7 provides an example of a collaborative in-class learning activity for the concept of Thermoregulation. In this activity, students consider why age groups have different risks for problems associated with thermoregulation. This collaborative work is assigned as an alternative to having an instructor present a slide listing risk factors. Alternatively, completion of this table may be used as a preclass assignment. In class, students can work in groups to compare and contrast and then develop a final table for presentation to the class.

Poster Fair

A variation on student presentations is the poster fair, a collaborative learning activity where student groups prepare and present posters to other members

---

BOX 6.7 ■ Risk Factor Assessment for the Concept of Thermoregulation

In your learning groups, complete the worksheet below by identifying common risk factors for thermoregulation problems across the life span.

Infants & Children	Adolescents/ Young Adults	Older Adults	Conclusion: How Are Risk Factors Similar? How Are They Different?

Adapted from TEACH for nurses for Giddens JF. *Concepts for Nursing Practice.* 2nd ed. St. Louis, MO: Elsevier; 2017.

BOX 6.8 ■ Collaborative Learning: Poster Fair for Health Promotion

In your learning groups, you will create a poster highlighting current evidence-based recommendations for your assigned health promotion topic. Be sure to include the parameters of the guidelines, particularly for specified population groups or persons with known risk factors, as appropriate. Include your reference. After groups have developed their posters, a poster fair will be held, and each group will share with others the key points for their topics.

---

of the class. Box 6.8 shows an example of a poster fair as a learning activity for the concept of *Health Promotion* with a focus on interventions. Student groups prepare posters for an in-class poster health fair outlining the current evidence for health promotion and health screening for various topics. Students learn from each other about the topics rather than from a faculty-driven presentation.

Concept Exemplars

Box 6.9 presents an example of a collaborative in-class learning activity in which students access the website of the Centers for Disease Control and Prevention to determine the most common types of infections in the United States (or their state) by age group. This activity links to the concept presentation and helps students gain an awareness of the broad range of exemplars they are likely to encounter in clinical practice. It is again important to reinforce the fact that instructors will not be teaching all the exemplars listed.

BOX 6.9 ■ Collaborative Learning: Exemplars of Infection

In your learning groups, visit the Centers for Disease Control and Prevention website and locate the statistics for infection prevalence by age group. Identify the 10 most commonly reported infections for each age group. Fill in your answers in the worksheet below and then determine what are similar or different.

Infants & Children	Adolescents/ Young Adults	Older Adults	Conclusions: How Are These Similar and Different?

Adapted from TEACH for nurses for Giddens JF. *Concepts for Nursing Practice.* 2nd ed. St. Louis, MO: Elsevier; 2017.

BOX 6.10 ■ Collaborative Learning: Concept Map of Interrelated Concepts

In your learning groups, discuss the relationship of the concepts listed below to the concept of *Development*. Draw a concept map showing the relationships.
- Culture
- Family Dynamics
- Genetics
- Nutrition
- Sensory Perception

Concept Maps

Student-developed concept maps provide a window into the mind of the student as he or she diagrams how concepts interrelate (Caputi and Blach, 2008). Students work in pairs or small groups to first develop simple maps and then expand those maps to demonstrate a growing complexity of concepts throughout the curriculum. For example, students work individually or in small groups to develop a concept map showing the relationship between *Development* and other concepts learned in the curriculum (Box 6.10). Students then discuss their rationale for the relationships made. Concept maps as a clinical-based strategy is discussed in Chapter 8.

Compare and Contrast

An excellent teaching strategy to promote thinking is comparing and contrasting similar situations or opposite ends of a spectrum. This technique can be used as

---

BOX 6.11 ■ Compare and Contrast: Degrees of Immunity

In your learning group, create a list of common symptoms and clinical findings associated with suppressed and exaggerated immunity and then discuss why each symptom or clinical finding occurs from a physiologic perspective.

Common Clinical Findings	
Suppressed Immunity	Exaggerated Immunity

Adapted from TEACH for nurses for Giddens JF. *Concepts for Nursing Practice.* 2nd ed. St. Louis, MO: Elsevier; 2017.

---

an in-class collaborative learning activity, or students can complete the task independently, after which the results can be used as discussion points in class. Box 6.11 provides an example of comparing and contrasting suppressed and exaggerated immune responses. Once the table is discussed, the information should be applied in class to several patient situations. The compare-and-contrast technique can be used for a number of different concepts in many different ways. As another example, compare and contrast can be used to highlight similarities and differences in a concept or exemplar based on age. Students are asked to compare and contrast the exemplar of asthma in a 70-year-old man and an 8-year-old girl. Such an activity not only provides an opportunity to gain a deeper understanding of the concept of gas exchange but also to gain an understanding of the variation in how the exemplar presents in different situations and the unique interrelated concepts for each of the two cases.

Questions That Promote Thinking

Faculty can challenge students to apply their thinking by presenting questions in the classroom for students to answer. Typically, this activity is performed using an audience response system. Once students have considered the question, before providing the answer, ask students to discuss their answers with a fellow student who answered differently. Studies have shown a positive correlation between learning with the use of clicker technology (Toothaker, 2018). The students should discuss their answers and the rationales for their answers. They will either convince their peer to change his or her answer or change their own answer based on new insights. Students engage in deep, meaningful learning as they are discussing their thinking processes with their peers. Of course, to be a conceptual learning method, the questions must be focused on concepts and not bits of information about the topic (Hardin and Richardson, 2012).

Summary

Teaching conceptually requires an intentional process to involve students in learning experiences that help them develop thinking skills that advance their ability to build a web of cognitive connections through conceptual understandings within the discipline of nursing. Developing a deep understanding of concepts requires the construction of cognitive frameworks through the lens of how nurses think. Purposeful, planned learning sessions for each concept in the curriculum are needed. The use of a standardized approach and the incorporation of the five principles (concepts, exemplars, context, link to previous understandings, and student engagement) underlie successful conceptual teaching. As evidenced by the variety of teaching strategies presented in this chapter, many teaching methods are used in a concept-based curriculum. Although only a sample of examples are presented, the underlying principles are that learning activities are deliberately planned with concepts being the major organizing factor, that the learning activities build on previous learning, and that learning is student-centered.

A primary purpose of inquiry-based learning strategies that focus on concepts is to build cognitive frameworks leading to enduring understanding and the ability to transfer knowledge to other situations and contexts. Several teaching strategies described in this chapter guide students through the process of thinking and reflecting, and help students develop skills in metacognition (an individual's understanding and awareness of their thought process). The volume of information nurses must process each day requires that they have skills in information management through cognitive recognition, interpretation, action, and reflection across multiple contexts. A systematic, formal process helping students develop these skills facilitates the formation of clinical judgment (McNelis et al., 2014; Tanner, 2006).

References

Anderson LW, Krathwohl DR. *A Taxonomy for Learning, Teaching, and Assessing: A Revision of Bloom's Taxonomy of Educational Objectives.* New York, NY: Longman; 2001.

Benner P, Sutphen M, Leonard V, et al. *Educating Nurses: A Call for Radical Transformation.* San Francisco, CA: Jossey-Bass; 2010.

Benner P, Tanner C, Chesla C. *Expertise in Nursing Practice: Caring, Clinical Judgment, and Ethics.* 2nd ed. New York, NY: Springer; 2009.

Brown PC, Roediger HL, McDaniel MA. *Make It Stick: The Science of Successful Learning.* Cambridge, MA: The Belknap Press of Harvard University Press; 2014.

Caputi L, Blach D. *Teaching Nursing Using Concept Maps.* Glen Ellyn, IL: DuPage Press; 2008.

Croteau SD, Howe LA, Timmons SM, Nilson L, Parker VG. Evaluation of the effectiveness of "The Village": a pharmacology education teaching strategy. *Nurs Educ Perspect.* 2011;32(5):338–341.

Curran R, Elfrink V, Mays B. Building a virtual community for nursing education: the town of Mirror Lake. *J Nurs Educ.* 2009;48(1):30–35.

Deane WH, Asselin M. Transitioning to concept-based teaching: a discussion of strategies and the use of Bridges change model. *J Nurs Educ Pract.* 2015;5(10):52–59.

del Bueno D. A crisis in critical thinking. *Nurs Educ Perspect.* 2005;26(5):278–282.

Dickison P, Luo X, Kim D, et al. Assessing higher order cognitive constructs by using an information-processing framework. *J Appl Test Technol.* 2016;17(1):1–19.

Giddens JF, Brady DP. Rescuing nursing education from content saturation: the case for a concept-based curriculum. *J Nurs Educ.* 2007;46(2):65–69.

Giddens JF. The neighborhood: a web-based platform to support conceptual teaching and learning. *Nurs Educ Perspect.* 2007;28(5):251–256.

Hardin PK, Richardson SJ. Teaching the concept curricula: theory and method. *J Nurs Educ.* 2012;51 (3):155–159.

Kavanagh JM, Sharpnack PA. Crisis in competency: a defining moment in nursing education. *Online J Issues Nurs.* 2021;26(1).

Kavanagh JM, Szweda C. A crisis in competency: the strategic and ethical imperative to assessing new graduate nurses' clinical reasoning. *Nurs Educ Perspect.* 2017;38(2):57–62.

Loyens S, Rikers R. Instruction based on inquiry. In: Mayer RE, Alexander PA, eds. *Handbook of Instruction on Learning and Instruction.* 2nd ed. New York, NY: Routledge; 2017.

McNelis AM, Ironside PM, Ebright PR, et al. Learning nursing practice: a multisite, multimethod investigation of clinical education. *J Nurs Regul.* 2014;4(4):30–35.

Murph PK, Wilkinson I, Soter AO, et al. Instruction based on discussion. In: Mayer RE, Alexander PA, eds. *Handbook of Instruction on Learning and Instruction.* 2nd ed. New York, NY: Routledge; 2017.

National Council of State Boards of Nursing. *Next Generation NCLEX Project*; 2021. https://www.ncsbn.org/next-generation-nclex.htm.

Repsha CL, Quinn BL, Peters AB. Implementing a concept-based nursing curriculum: a review of the literature. *Teach Learn Nurs.* 2020;15:66–71. https://doi.org/10.1016/j.teln.2019.09.006.

Schunk DH. *Learning Theories: An Educational Perspective.* 6th ed. Upper Saddle River, NJ: Pearson; 2012.

Scheckel M. Designing courses and learning experiences. In: Billings DM, Halstead JA, eds. *Teaching in Nursing: A Guide for Faculty.* 5th ed. St. Louis MO: Elsevier; 2016.

Sportsman S, Pleasant T. Concept-based curricula: State of the innovation. *Teaching and Learning in Nursing.* 2017;12:195–200.

Slavin RE. Instruction based on cooperative learning. In: Mayer RE, Alexander PA, eds. *Handbook of Instruction on Learning and Instruction.* 2nd ed. New York, NY: Routledge; 2017.

Takase M, Yoshida I. The relationship between the types of learning approaches used by undergraduate nursing students and their academic achievement: a systematic review and meta-analysis. *J Prof Nurs.* 2021;37:836–845.

Tanner CA. Thinking like a nurse: a research model of clinical judgement in nursing. *J Nurs Edu.* 2006;45(6):204–211.

Toothaker R. Millennial's perspective of clicker technology in a nursing classroom: a mixed methods research study. *Nurse Educ Today.* 2018;62:80–84.

Walsh M. Narrative pedagogy and simulation: future directions for nursing education. *Nurse Educ Pract.* 2011;11:216–219.

CHAPTER 7

Concept-Based Instruction for Clinical Education

Clinical teaching and learning represent important components of nursing education by enabling students to apply knowledge, concepts, and clinical skills learned in the classroom to the practice setting. Clinical learning activities provide the opportunity to extend and deepen students' conceptual understandings because they directly experience concepts associated with the nursing discipline as they appear in practice. Astute students will notice that concepts take on a multitude of variations across clinical practice areas and across a variety of patients; this awareness is necessary for developing more complex cognitive patterns of thinking that lead to clinical judgment. However, being in a clinical setting does not automatically result in deepened conceptual understandings; clinical education must be intentionally designed to achieve this outcome. This chapter provides an overview of planning and implementing conceptual teaching strategies in the clinical setting.

Traditional Clinical Education

The primary learning activity in a traditional clinical education model is for nursing students to provide total patient care to an assigned patient (or patients) in parallel with nursing staff. There is an emphasis on clock hours spent in clinical, clinical skill development, preclinical paperwork, and written assignments to be submitted after clinical; often there is a disconnect between clinical learning and learning in didactic courses. This model, which has been the standard for more than 50 years (despite changes to education and health care), has largely been based on a "learning to practice" perspective. In other words, it is based on the assumption that learning occurs as a result of performing that care. However, the effectiveness of this model has been increasingly questioned. Shockingly, recent systematic reviews to examine evidence for current clinical education practices found no evidence to support traditional clinical education models (Leighton et al., 2021, 2022)! Such findings support and add to concerns raised a decade ago (Institute of Medicine [IOM], 2010; Tanner, 2010).

Many limitations in traditional clinical education have been identified. For one thing, it is difficult for the clinical instructor to effectively facilitate learning with a large group of students who are all providing total patient care. Also, the type of learning experiences students gain is dependent on patient acuity and the times students are in the clinical setting. Furthermore, the presence of multiple students simultaneously performing total patient care places an unnecessary burden on nursing staff within the clinical area. Traditional clinical education has been described as "education by random opportunity" (LeFlore et al., 2007, p. 170)—underscoring the point that it represents limited consistency. Because typical activities of students are directed at patient care, this model essentially misplaces the student in the role of a nurse as opposed to the role of learner.

In a study evaluating outcomes associated with traditional clinical education, researchers reported that (1) students had too much "down time"; (2) too much time was focused on performing repetitive tasks that do not result in new learning; and (3) too little time was focused on developing higher-order thinking skills (Ironside and McNelis, 2010). In a subsequent study, McNelis and colleagues reported that higher-level thinking was not a primary focus in prelicensure nursing clinical education and that thinking at the application and analysis level was not rewarded (McNelis et al., 2014). Although students spend a large amount of time in the clinical setting, many of those clinical hours fail to result in productive learning. Faculty report spending most of their time supervising students in hands-on procedures, leaving little time to focus on fostering the development of clinical reasoning skills (IOM, 2010; McNelis et al., 2014). It was pointed out more than a decade ago that "not all learning objectives require students to practice total patient care" (Gaberson and Oermann, 2007, p. 95). Moreover, not everything that needs to be learned can be effectively accomplished when providing total patient care. Although still prevalent, traditional approaches are slowly giving way to more contemporary clinical education practices.

Contemporary Concept-Based Clinical Education

New trends in clinical education have emerged to better prepare students for entry-level clinical practice. A "practice to learn" perspective reframes contemporary clinical education as a component of the learning process and aligns with the clinical learning that is essential and desired in a concept-based curriculum. In the clinical setting, concepts come alive through a multitude of situations and activities. Concept-based learning activities (CBLAs) are intentionally designed and incorporated into clinical courses as part of an overall curriculum plan. Clinical experiences serve as additional exemplars on which to extend and deepen conceptual understandings. Competencies associated with selected concepts can be used as measurable clinical outcomes associated with clinical education and practice. Advocates for changes to clinical education emphasize the need for deepening understanding of key concepts and application of thinking to develop clinical judgment (Caputi, 2018; Giddens and Brady, 2007; Jessee, 2018; Lasater and Nielsen, 2009a; Nielsen, 2016; Nielsen et al., 2021; Oermann et al., 2018; Tanner, 2006). Contemporary clinical education allows students to gain a deep understanding of concepts through the interaction and application in a clinical context. Tanner (2010) proposed three foci for clinical education to better prepare students for safe practice: (1) deepening and extending theoretical knowledge and learning how key concepts are exemplified in practice; (2) developing clinical judgment using a variety of thinking skills and strategies; and (3) developing an understanding of the culture of health care and nursing and how the health care system functions, especially as it relates to the patient, the nurse, and interactions with other interprofessional health care providers. Thus, the contemporary model of clinical education not only supports conceptual learning but also supports student-centered learning with an emphasis on communication, collaboration, peer or group learning, and the development of clinical reasoning and clinical judgment.

OUTCOMES OF CONCEPT-BASED CLINICAL EDUCATION

Schools that adopt a concept-based curriculum share a similar perspective regarding the approach for education. Several contextual factors that influence decisions made within each program (such as type of nursing program, setting of the program, and resources) make each curriculum unique—thus faculty make decisions about the approach for clinical education that aligns with the curriculum. Although the clinical education plan is driven by unique curriculum outcomes, the three learning domains—cognitive, psychomotor, and affective—underlie learning outcomes and are foundational to conceptual learning activities. Focus areas for each domain in clinical teaching are presented in Table 7.1. Faculty should consider these domains as a key part of the overall clinical education design.

Competencies represent another important component of clinical education in a concept-based curriculum. In Chapter 2, it was noted that a competency is an outcomes-based statement of what is expected of the learner as it relates to a concept and/or domain. A competency incorporates knowledge, skills, and attitudes as an expression of performance expectation that is observable and measurable. Thus, an intentional plan is devised to ensure that students have multiple learning experiences with concepts in a variety of situations and complexity, providing several opportunities to demonstrate the associated competencies.

SETTINGS FOR CLINICAL EDUCATION

Contemporary clinical education models use a variety of settings for clinical learning experiences. Historically, clinical nursing education has predominantly

TABLE 7.1 ■ **Domains of Learning in Clinical Education**

Cognitive Domain	Psychomotor Domain	Affective Domain
• Problem Solving	• Psychomotor Skills	• Professional Roles
• Critical Thinking	• Interpersonal Skills	• Accountability
• Clinical Judgment & Decision Making	• Organizational Skills	• Ethics
		• Values

taken place in acute care, inpatient settings where a faculty member oversees a group of nursing students who provide care to one or more assigned patients. This setting remains an important component of clinical education. However, health care delivery occurs in multiple settings and, thus, the settings where professional nurses practice and are needed have evolved. For these reasons, a variety of settings for clinical education should be incorporated into the clinical education plan.

Patient Care Environments

The need and expectation for the diversification of clinical education settings is reflected in two prominent reports. The American Association of Colleges of Nursing (AACN) revised *Essentials* specifically recommends that all students have clinical experiences within four distinct "spheres" of current and future areas of healthcare delivery—including health promotion/wellness; chronic disease care; regenerative, acute care; and hospice/palliative care (American Association of Colleges of Nursing [AACN], 2021). This recommendation was influenced by Lipstein and colleagues who described the workforce needs for 21st century healthcare (Lipstein et al., 2016). Diversification of nursing practice settings is also noted by the National Academics of Sciences, Engineering, and Medicine (NASEM) in their consensus study report *The Future of Nursing: 2020–2030: Charting a Path to Achieve Health Equity* (National Academies of Sciences, Engineering, and Medicine [NASEM], 2021). Specifically, the NASEM noted a need for more nurses prepared for practice in a variety of community-based settings, public health (including disaster response), home health care, telehealth settings, and other innovative models of community-based care.

Currently, many common healthcare delivery settings (such as outpatient clinics, perioperative settings, nursing homes, extended care facilities, and hospice and palliative care settings) tend to be underused for clinical teaching. The evolution of contemporary clinical education has led to the expansion of clinical learning to diverse sites within the community (such as childcare and early education program, schools, summer camps, wellness centers) and international opportunities (Oermann et al., 2018). Most nursing concepts are not setting-specific; thus the application of curriculum concepts across health care settings provides a deeper understanding of the concept through multiple clinical contexts. As Oermann et al. (2018) point out, "nursing care can be learned wherever students have contact with patients" (p. 35).

CBLAs can easily be designed to occur in all health care settings described, with an emphasis on learning within the context of the clinical site and with patients typically associated within the site. Faculty must be willing to reimagine clinical education to optimize this opportunity. Obviously, clinical sites must provide the ability for students to meet the learning outcomes of the course, thus, the type of patients and care provided within the site are two important factors. A positive environment that is inviting to students and committed to supporting student learning is just as important. Nurses within the clinical site are also integral to the students' learning, thus, gaining their support and cooperation is essential. Staff nurses who are accustomed to supporting student learning in a traditional clinical education model may need additional reinforcement of the learning to take place so as to avoid confusion and facilitate cooperation.

Laboratory and Simulation Learning Environment

In addition to patient care settings, the clinical laboratory and simulation laboratory represent other important areas to conduct clinical education. Learning in laboratory and simulation settings provides students with meaningful learning experiences for clinical skill development and scenario-based learning. In a concept-based curriculum, a combination of low- and high-fidelity experiences is framed around applicable concepts. The term *fidelity* refers to how closely something resembles reality. Low fidelity means the experience is somewhat close to reproducing what is real; high fidelity means the experience is very close to reproducing what is real.

Conceptual teaching approaches within simulation can be accomplished by developing scenarios with an emphasis on a concept, or by creating complex scenarios involving multiple concepts. As an example, if there is a desire that all students have a simulation experience caring for a patient with impaired perfusion, simulation scenarios can be developed to feature a desired exemplar of impaired perfusion (such as myocardial infarction or heart failure). If time allows, a series of simulation activities featuring different exemplars of the same concept could be completed, allowing students to experience variations in the concept, not only in the type of health condition, but also the age of patient, or the patient care setting. For advanced students, simulation experiences featuring *concept clusters* (meaning a group of interrelated concepts that commonly occur in clinical situations) provide the opportunity for students to gain experience managing patients with multiple needs and in their determining priorities. Simulations featuring concept clusters represent another way to provide integrated learning experiences and to assess learning outcomes.

A second opportunity to incorporate conceptual learning in a simulation is during debriefing. Because simulation provides students with clinical experiences that are close to a real-world experience, the same type of thinking that is taught and used in the patient care clinical setting should be incorporated in simulation. Guidance during debriefing should focus the thinking process for clinical decision making as it relates to the concept. Box 7.1 provides examples of elements related to conceptual thinking that can be used as a guide during simulation debriefing.

TYPES OF CLINICAL LEARNING

Conceptual learning in the clinical setting is achieved through a variety of learning experiences and settings through CBLAs. Intentionally designed CBLAs integrated within *total patient care* and *focused clinical activities* provide structure, increase the consistency of clinical education experiences, and ensure the application of concepts in the clinical setting. These two types of learning activities are not mutually exclusive—meaning that in some cases a student may complete a

> **BOX 7.1 ▪ Sample Questions for Simulation Debriefing**
>
> **Debriefing after a High-fidelity Simulation Experience**
> - What were the primary concepts of concern in this patient situation?
> - What were the assessment findings that you considered highest priority? How did this affect your decisions and the priority for the nursing actions you completed?
> - Did the patient respond as you expected? If not, what surprised you? Why do you believe the patient responded in that manner?
> - What did you do well? Reflecting on this experience, what could you have done differently to be more effective in the patient care? In what areas do you think you need further practice?
> - What other concepts are often present in a clinical situation such as this?

focused clinical activity (FCA) while also involved in a total patient care experience. The Oregon Consortium for Nursing Education was an early proponent of purposefully embedding a variety of structured clinical learning experiences (including direct clinical care experiences, concept-based experiences, case-based experiences, skill-based experiences, and integrative experiences) into a curriculum model (Gubrud-Howe and Schoessler, 2008).

Total Patient Care

Total patient care refers to a clinical assignment where the student is responsible for planning, implementing, and evaluating care for one or more patients. This type of learning requires the students to integrate multiple aspects of care into the clinical experience and demonstrate competence in patient care management; for this reason, total patient care is especially valuable for students in an immersion capstone clinical experience. The instructor or preceptor determines what level of care interventions the student will do during total patient care activities; this is largely driven by care practices in the clinical site, and level of student. Variations include assigning more than one patient to a student or assigning one or more patients to more than one student (student teams). In a concept-based curriculum, concept application is incorporated through written assignments (such as a care plan or concept map), discussions with faculty, and clinical conference presentations.

Focused Clinical Activities

An *FCA* is a structured learning experience designed to support various aspects of clinical learning to fulfill specific course or program learning outcomes and/or competencies. In a concept-based curriculum, the focus of learning is based on one or more concepts in a specific clinical context (Nielsen, 2009). Depending on the design, FCAs involve direct interaction with patients and can be completed by students independently or in groups in any clinical learning setting. On occasion, an FCA may occur through shadowing or observational experiences to develop a greater understanding of concepts associated with professional nursing practice, and interprofessional practice (IPP).

MISCONCEPTIONS AND CLARIFICATIONS

Misconception: All students within a clinical learning group should be involved in the same clinical learning activities on any given day to maintain consistency among the learners and to avoid confusing the nursing staff in the clinical areas.

Clarification: All students within a clinical group may complete the same clinical learning activities over the course of a semester or term, but students may be involved in different learning activities on the same day. Some students may be assigned to total patient care while others may complete a focused clinical activity assignment.

Designing Concept-Based Learning Activities for the Clinical Setting

The design of CBLAs was previously discussed in Chapter 6, in the context of classroom/didactic teaching. However, CBLAs are also designed for clinical education. Contemporary clinical education is intentionally planned as part of the overall curriculum design by considering the learning outcomes, competencies, the desired learning domains, desired concepts, the level of the learner, and the setting where clinical learning will occur. Ideally, faculty develop a specific curriculum-wide plan for how CBLAs are incorporated into each clinical course. In a concept-based curriculum the clinical learning focuses on the application of the concept or concepts in a specific clinical context; concepts are further incorporated into written assignments, discussions with the faculty member, and in clinical conference.

CREATING A LESSON PLAN

Developing a lesson plan for clinical teaching is similar to the planning that underlies classroom-based teaching. Specific clinical assignments are incorporated into the course syllabus and course materials so that students have a clear understanding of what is expected of them. This also leads to increased consistency and accountability among faculty, particularly when multiple sections of the same clinical course are taught by different faculty. In addition to curriculum outcomes, course objectives, and competencies, factors used to plan CBLAs include the level/experience of the student, the type of clinical site(s), and the course placement (cycle) within the curriculum. Learning outcomes, concepts, related competencies, expected student activities, and deliverables completed throughout the clinical experience should also be considered as part of the lesson plan. Use of a standardized lesson plan template for clinical learning helps achieve consistency from a curricular standpoint. Elements to include in clinical lesson planning are shown in Box 7.2.

Another important consideration is that in a contemporary clinical education model, students within a clinical group may be involved in different learning activities in different locations and on the same or other days. In other words,

---

BOX 7.2 ■ Elements of a Concept-Based Learning Activity Lesson Plan for Clinical Education

- Activity name
- Concept(s) under study
- Learning outcomes and/or competency
- Specific activities students complete
- Role of faculty to facilitate learning
- Method of evaluation (written assignment, presentation, etc.)

---

some students may be doing total patient care and other students may be doing FCAs. Depending on the complexity, an FCA may be completed by an individual student or within student teams. This approach allows for greater efficiency in the use of clinical sites with limited capacity.

ASSIGNMENTS

Assignments are an essential element of the clinical lesson plan. The purpose of a clinical assignment is to promote the understanding of concepts and other information. promote thinking and clinical judgment, promote reflection on the experience (including an exploration of students' feelings, beliefs, or attitudes), and to provide a mechanism for feedback and evaluation. In a concept-based curriculum, concepts are planned as a component of the clinical assignment. There are many types of assignments that can be incorporated into CBLAs. Driving factors for determining the type of assignment include the clinical site, the type of learning activity, and the desired learning outcome. Common clinical assignments include a concept map, a concept analysis, case study, case presentation, nursing care plan, development of a teaching plan, reflective journal, short written assignments, guided worksheets, compare and contrast assignments, evidence-based practice assignments, and assessment assignments. A few of these assignments are discussed further below.

Concept Map

A concept map is a diagram of key concepts in the context of patient care or related to a situation, each of which shows key relationships between the concepts. It allows students to explore the health conditions or factors affecting the patient and translate these into appropriate representative concepts. This process fosters the integration of multiple concepts into cognitive understanding; further, this strategy is credited with increasing student critical thinking and metacognition (Alfayoumi, 2019; Rahnama and Mardani-Hamooleh, 2017; Senita, 2008; Taylor and Littleton-Keamey, 2011). Concept maps can be used in the clinical setting as an individual assignment or as a collaborative assignment for both total patient care and FCAs. There are a number of ways a concept map assignment can be created (Daley et al., 2016); thus, faculty will need to develop parameters for such an assignment. Fig. 7.1 shows an example of a concept map assignment.

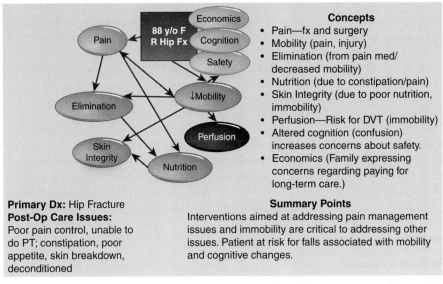

Fig. 7.1 The concept map is a common concept-based teaching strategy used in nursing. *DVT,* Deep vein thrombosis; *PT,* physical therapy.

Concept Analysis

As an assignment for learners, a concept analysis is an excellent way to reinforce conceptual understandings. This is not to be confused with a formal concept analysis in the research context, which involves an intense review and study of the literature. In an educational context, students conduct a review of what is known about a concept as it presents in an assigned patient (or patients) or a situation within the clinical environment to reinforce the commonalities of the concept. The analysis can take the form of a clinical presentation and/or a clinical written paper.

Case Study and Case Presentation With Conceptual Focus

A case study is a written assignment with a focus on a single patient, family, setting, or situation. Students provide a written narrative of the events in the context of the major concepts involved following a template or assignment guide. In some cases, a concept map may be created to accompany the case study. A case presentation is similar but is more of an oral presentation—often done in a clinical seminar or during patient rounds.

Nursing Care Plan

A nursing care plan has been used for a number of years as an assignment in the clinical area. A typical care plan approach includes a patient assessment to identify nursing diagnoses, set care goals, determine appropriate interventions and then evaluate the interventions. These elements are presented in a column format, with each diagnosis addressed independently in a linear format. Students prioritize three to five diagnoses for each care plan—and, more often than not, the nursing diagnoses represent concepts. The value of a care plan is that it helps the student learn the nursing process. Although care plans can still be used in a concept-based curriculum, critics suggest that a care plan limits thinking, approaches problems in a linear approach, and fails to address the reality of interrelated problems. Furthermore, the usefulness of care plans for stimulating higher-level thinking has come into question (Oermann et al., 2018).

Teaching Plan

A teaching plan has been a common clinical assignment for years. In a concept-based curriculum, students apply relevant teaching and learning concepts to create a health teaching plan for a patient, family, or community. Although specifics of assignments may vary, a teaching plan typically includes a learner assessment, objectives, developing content, and consideration of appropriate teaching strategies for the target learner. These plans can be completed by students individually or as a collaborative assignment.

Reflective Journal

A reflective journal fosters reflective thinking, which is an underlying component for developing clinical judgment (Lasater and Nielsen, 2009b). This is typically an independent assignment where students think about the concepts involved in the context of the care they provided or the situation observed and then reflect on questions posed by the faculty member.

MISCONCEPTIONS AND CLARIFICATIONS

Misconception: Designing concept-based teaching strategies for the clinical environment is challenging because the concepts must be present in the clinical environment in a similar order as concepts are presented in the curriculum.

Clarification: A concept-based approach allows greater flexibility for learning compared to a traditional content-focused curriculum. Nearly all nursing concepts presented in a nursing curriculum are in all clinical sites every day! For this reason, matching concepts in the clinical area to the sequencing of concepts in the curriculum is not an issue. As students learn concepts in didactic courses, specific concept exemplars are presented in class. The clinical environment represents a multitude of other exemplars of the same concept to extend and deepen learning. In other words, the clinical environment allows students to see how that concept applies in other ways.

Exemplars of Concept-Based Learning Activities in the Clinical Setting

Conceptual learning in the clinical areas involves making purposeful connections to curricular concepts discussed in didactic courses. The large majority of concepts are evident in all clinical areas, so the only limits to learning are those placed by the faculty. Additionally, students will encounter clinical situations and patients representing important curricular concepts they have not yet formally learned about. This issue is no different than any other curriculum model. Faculty should plan to help students make connections to these concepts through other means. In all likelihood, the students probably have had some level of exposure or awareness to many things before having a formal concept presentation. For this reason, faculty should try to not overthink or be too prescriptive regarding conceptual learning in the clinical environment.

Concepts are represented by a multitude of exemplars, so the goal is to help students learn from any situation. For example, if the students have studied the concept of *Gas Exchange* in the classroom, every patient encounter is an opportunity to deepen their understanding of *Gas Exchange*. Considering that *Gas Exchange* ranges from optimal to significant impairment of gas exchange and that the concept is evident in all humans across the life span and in every clinical setting, a learning activity in *Gas Exchange* does not require assigning a student to a patient in respiratory distress. Students can learn about *Gas Exchange* from any patient.

As discussed earlier in this chapter, faculty develop and implement CBLA lesson plans for clinical learning. This leads to greater consistency among clinical groups and an improved ability to track expected clinical learning outcomes. Examples of CBLAs for the clinical environment are provided in the sections that follow.

SAFETY

Safety is a core concept that should be intentionally incorporated into clinical learning. An example of a CBLA focused on the concept of *Safety* is presented in Box 7.3. Once completed, students should incorporate what they learned about safety on subsequent clinical days as part of the individual student's patient care experience. In other words, this is not a "one and done" experience—rather, this type of thinking should be continuously applied to learn the nuances and salient features within each patient context and within each type of health care environment.

MOBILITY

Box 7.4 is an example of a CBLA associated with the concept of *Mobility*. During this activity, students assess an assigned patient and compare findings to those learned from the concept-presentation or literature regarding the mobility concept. Students determine whether the level of mobility is expected and

---

BOX 7.3 ■ Concept-Based Learning Activity for the Concept of Safety

Title: National Patient Safety Goals in the Clinical Setting
Concept: Safety
Learning outcome: Assess how the National Patient Safety Goals are applied in the clinical setting.
Activities to complete:
- Pre-Clinical Preparation: (1) Locate and download the current *National Patient Safety Goals* from The Joint Commission website. Review the goals (simplified version) in each of the areas (ambulatory care, behavioral health care, etc.) and notice commonalities across clinical sites. Bring a copy of the goals that most closely link with the clinical site you will be in. (2) Locate and download the clinical worksheet for this CBLA.
- Review the National Safety Goals and find evidence that actions are being taken within the clinical site to meet the goals and protocol. Specifically, address the following questions:
  - For each goal, describe the actions you observed nurses and other health care providers take to meet the goal. Also note if you saw inconsistency in practice.
  - Were there any goals you were unable to assess? If so, which ones? For goals you were unable to directly assess, discuss with nurses in the care environment how they would ensure achievement of those goals. Compare their answers to national safety guidelines.
  - What factors regarding the environment indicate that these safety goals are being met and what factors regarding the environment indicate a need for change so the safety goals can be met?

Assessment of learning: Complete and submit the worksheet for this assignment located in your course materials and address the questions listed above. Be prepared to share your experiences with the clinical group during debriefing in post-conference.

CBLA, Concept-based learning activity.
Adapted from: Caputi L. *Think Like a Nurse: A Handbook.* Rolling Meadows, IL, Windy City Publishers; 2018.

BOX 7.4 ■ Concept-Based Learning Activity for the Concept of Mobility

Title: Evaluating Patient Activity Level
Concept: Mobility
Learning outcome: Assess the activity level of an assigned patient and identify appropriate nursing interventions.
Related competencies: Integrate assessment skills; identify actual or potential problems; demonstrate clinical judgment to ensure accurate and safe care.
Activities to complete:
- Collect the following data that may affect activity level for your assigned patient. These include: age, gender, presenting health condition and other preexisting conditions, current medications, presence of pain or discomfort, and recent procedures, if applicable.

BOX 7.4 ■ Concept-Based Learning Activity for the Concept of Mobility (continued)

- Conduct an assessment (including an assessment of the patient's gait, balance, posture, and ease of movement, if possible). Also, be sure to ask the patient about their typical level of activity and any recent changes.
- Consider the data listed above and identify actual or potential effects these may have on the patient's activity level. Also, identify risk factors for impaired mobility.

Assessment of learning:

- During post-conference, present the patient(s) in a case format and incorporate the following guiding questions: (1) Is the level of activity expected and acceptable? Why? Why not? (2) What level of activity can be expected for the patient without causing harm? (3) If the patient is not able to engage in the expected level of activity, what actions should be taken? What consequences could occur?
- Complete and submit the worksheet for this assignment located in your course materials.

---

acceptable, as well as identify risks. By collecting the appropriate data and then making interpretations and inferences about those data, students arrive at conclusions that guide actions in clinical practice. The process of analysis, interpretation, and decision-making helps to facilitate clinical judgment.

PERFUSION

Perfusion is a concept that can be applied to any patient in any setting—because students can learn about perfusion from people who have optimal perfusion, as well as impaired perfusion. Box 7.5 is an example of a CBLA for the concept of perfusion that is intended to deepen students' recognition of how perfusion presents in the clinical setting in a variety of patients. Specifically, students assess individuals to determine whether they have optimal or impaired perfusion and assess risk factors for impaired perfusion. They also evaluate the care to determine which interventions (if any) support perfusion and the effectiveness of those interventions.

HEALTH CARE SYSTEMS

A number of concepts link to health care systems such as Health Care Organizations, Health Care Economics, Health Policy, Ethics, Safety, Health Care Quality, and Technology and Informatics. The traditional model for clinical instruction places the students in patient' rooms for the majority of the time they are in the clinical setting, and, thus, their learning tends to be limited to the perspective of the individual nurse and perhaps the unit of care. Students have often missed opportunities to learn about these concepts on a systems level. Spector

---

BOX 7.5 ■ Concept-Based Learning Activity for the Concept of Perfusion

Title: Perfusion Assessment and Analysis
Concept: Perfusion
Competencies: Retrieves appropriate information from the health record; conducts a health assessment; clinical judgment
Activities to complete:
- Conduct an in-depth assessment and analysis of perfusion on three assigned patients. This includes a review of a health record, patient assessment, and review of care.
- Gather and record the following information for each patient to organize your thoughts.

Relevant Data	Patient 1	Patient 2	Patient 3
Gender, age			
Existing health conditions			
Data from health record			
Data from health assessment			
Interventions to support perfusion (if applicable)			
Conclusion: optimal, impaired, or at risk for impaired perfusion?			

Analysis: What common elements of the concept of perfusion exist among all three patients? What differences exist and why?
Assessment of learning: Complete and submit the worksheet table and analysis for this assignment located in your course materials.

---

and Echternacht (2011) report that a number of studies have cited actual errors and near misses that have resulted from a lack of familiarity with the workplace environment. Box 7.6 provides an example of a CBLA focusing on the concepts of Health Care Quality and Safety. In this example, the students review the concepts in the context of medication administration from the perspective of the individual nurse, the unit of care, and at the system level. The importance of safe administration of medications cannot be overemphasized. However, because of time constraints, many faculty focus exclusively on the actual psychomotor skill of administering medications. Although psychomotor skills are important, students completing a learning activity such as this gain great insight regarding the entire process of medication administration. Students learn ways to not only avoid errors in medication administration but to identify potential problems and work to resolve them before an error is made.

BOX 7.6 ■ Concept-Based Learning Activity: Health Care Systems, Quality, and Safety

Title: Best Practices for Medication Administration and Error Prevention

Concepts: Health Care Systems; Quality; Safety

Competencies: Incorporate evidence-based approach for medication administration; Examine principles and processes to reduce error.

Activities to complete:

1. Follow a nurse and specifically observe the administration of medications. Watch and note every step of the process, including the process for new medication orders, the processing of the medication order into the system, reviewing the order, retrieving the medication, administration of the medication, documentation, and observing for evidence of the effects. Be sure to also notice how the nurse manages multiple patients, resources used for safe medication delivery, and the system used to keep track of time for medication delivery.

2. Ask clarifying questions to learn as much as you can regarding the process. Discuss with the nurse the most common challenges associated with medication management. Also talk with a pharmacist to gain an alternative perspective.

3. Create an illustration or flow chart to represent medication administration process, incorporating system factors and unit of care factors.

Assessment of learning:

- Share your experiences with the clinical group during post-conference. Describe things observed to ensure safe medication delivery. Also discuss areas where potential errors could occur and measures that could reduce the possibility of error.

- Write a two-page reflection paper on your experience, including things you observed such as roles of various team members, evidence of adherence to medication administration protocol, areas where errors could have occurred, what you learned from the experience, and how you will incorporate what you learned into your practice moving forward. Submit your flow chart with your paper.

CLINICAL SKILL DEVELOPMENT

Clinical nursing skills are an important component of nursing education. These are often taught initially in a nursing skills laboratory setting and/or they may be integrated into courses throughout the nursing program and taught as part of a concept overview. Regardless, students should gain confidence performing clinical skills correctly, they should understand the context of the skill as a nursing intervention, and they should understand how the skill factors into patient care through a conceptual lens. For this reason, faculty should be intentional about planning opportunities for students to discover linkages between nursing skills and concepts. Students continue to practice skills in the patient care areas under the supervision of the clinical faculty and may be linked to expected clinical competencies.

BOX 7.7 ■ Concept-Based Learning Activity to Support Skill Development

Title: Recognition of Concepts through Assessment

Concept: Patient-Centered Care

Competencies: Complete a history and physical assessment; Recognize actual or potential health problems.

Activities to complete:
- Conduct a history and physical assessment on your assigned patient. After completing the assessment, document your findings in the patient health record.
- Based on the assessment findings, consider the following:
  1. What are the top three to five priority concepts identified?
  2. In what way do the assessment findings reflect concept attributes and criteria?
  3. How are the medical conditions or health concerns related to these concepts?
  4. Are additional data needed to better understand the conditions or concerns?
  5. What interventions are currently being done and what additional interventions should be considered?

Assessment of learning:
- Complete and submit the worksheet provided for this assignment.
- Include a reflection on how this assignment extended your understanding of the concepts and your assessment competence.

Patient assessment—which includes conducting a history and physical examination—is usually introduced in the nursing skills laboratory and students continue to learn and develop these skills in patient care areas. To help move students from a task-oriented approach of assessment to thinking like a nurse, students require deliberate guidance. Box 7.7 provides an example of CBLA focused on patient assessment and the recognition/identification of priority concepts. The patient data sheet organizes the assessment data conceptually; thus, a deep understanding of concepts facilitates the determination of individual patient needs.

As students advance, they should be able to conduct an assessment and identify patient needs without any prior knowledge of the patient or the patient's condition. This enhances competence and confidence to independently identify issues and problems, and then gain clarification regarding findings based on existing health records and reports from other health care providers.

INTERPROFESSIONAL EDUCATION

Nurses represent the largest group of health care professionals involved in the delivery of health care. Effective delivery of comprehensive, efficient, and high-quality health care depends on high-functioning health care teams. The hallmarks of effective health care teams are reflected in the competencies proposed by the Interprofessional Education Collaborative (IPEC) and include interprofessional teamwork and team-based practice, interprofessional communication practices, and values and ethics for IPP (which includes an awareness and appreciation for unique roles, responsibilities, and contributions made by all members of the health care team) (Interprofessional Education Collaborative [IPEC], 2016). Nursing education must prepare nursing students to work within interprofessional health care teams. Because interprofessional teamwork is learned in the practice setting (Durkin and Feinn, 2017), intentional interprofessional education (IPE) learning experiences should be designed and incorporated in the clinical education curriculum based on the IPEC core competencies.

The IPEC competencies link to several professional nursing and health care concepts (*Collaboration, Teamwork, Communication, Ethics, Care Coordination*), thus, there is great opportunity for IPE to be gained through clinical learning activities featuring these concepts. These should not be approached as an "add-on" to the curriculum, but rather incorporated as clinical teaching strategies (Oermann et al., 2018). Thus, there should not be an expectation that all students have identical IPE experiences. Ideally, students will share their experiences and reflections in a post-clinical conference. Specific learning activities can include simulation experiences (described previously) with students from other health care disciplines, observation experiences, clinical rounding, and patient planning meetings.

Experiences in Areas of Exemplary Interprofessional Practice

Students can gain very robust IPE experiences through experiences in clinical sites where strong IPP exists. Nursing faculty will first identify exemplary clinical sites where IPP occurs for optimal student learning. Areas where strong teamwork is typically seen include perioperative and surgery, rehabilitation hospitals and clinics, and mental health services. Many other clinical sites, particularly in community settings addressing health care access for the underserved, or those addressing the health care needs of individuals with complex multimorbid conditions, also tend to have strong IPP. Box 7.8 provides an example of a CBLA using observation experience for IPE.

Patient Rounding or Patient Care Conferencing

Another learning activity to address IPE includes interprofessional patient rounding. This type of experience involves multiple health care professionals (such as physicians, nurses, pharmacists, dieticians, social workers, case managers) discussing each patient assigned to the team and working together to develop a plan of care. Although true rounding is most commonly seen in inpatient areas, interprofessional rounding may also occur in a modified format (such as a team conference) in other settings. Nursing faculty must gain the permission and cooperation from the clinical team leader conducting rounds (or the unit where the patient rounds will occur) for the student to participate as a team member in the patient rounds. Students prepare for the experience by becoming familiar with the patients on whom rounds will occur. The students should be prepared to present and discuss the patients during rounding from a nursing

---

BOX 7.8 ■ Concept-Based Learning Activity for Interprofessional Education

Title: Interactions and Teamwork in Interprofessional Practice

Concepts: Collaboration, Communication

Competencies: Communicate effectively with members of the health care team; Collaborate with other health care team professionals.

Activities to complete:

Observe the clinical environment with an emphasis on the interactions and collaboration of the various members of the health care team. As appropriate, ask clarifying questions to learn as much as you can regarding how the various team members interact and work together. Specifically assess and make note of the following:

- The health care setting, including the type of care provided and types of patients seen
- The health care professionals represented
- The roles and expertise of each member of the health care team
- Contributions of each team member in the delivery of care
- Patterns of communication between team members
- Examples of effective teamwork
- Challenges experienced and how the team worked together for solutions

Assessment of learning: Write a two-page reflection paper addressing the things you were specifically asked to observe (above). Describe your impressions of the benefits and challenges working within the health care team and the level of respect observed among various health team members and the impact on health care outcomes. Describe how your assessment aligns with the concepts of collaboration and communication.

---

perspective. Students should have an opportunity to share their experience in a post-clinical conference focusing on their impressions regarding how well the team collaborated, contributions made by various members of the team, and how members of the team collaborated in the decision-making process. Faculty should also consider asking the student to complete a written assignment based on the experience.

Faculty Role/Expectations in Clinical Education

In most nursing programs, clinical courses are taught by both full-time faculty and part-time or adjunct faculty. A general challenge associated with clinical education is maintaining consistency and quality in the clinical learning experience—this becomes an even greater challenge if faculty are unfamiliar with a concept-based curriculum. It is critical that the adoption of a conceptual approach includes a transition and faculty development plan for instructors (Giddens and Brady, 2007; Hendricks and Wangerin, 2017; Repsha et al.,

2020; Sportsman and Pleasant, 2017). Professional development is discussed further in Chapter 9.

The delivery of excellent concept-based clinical instruction requires that the instructor must have expertise in the clinical area he or she is assigned to teach, understand the conceptual approach, and follow the teaching plan for the clinical course, which includes ensuring that students complete the various CBLAs and provide an evaluation of student learning. Additionally, the instructor should be perceived as approachable (especially by the students), build rapport with nurses in the clinical setting, have excellent interpersonal skills, and possess clinical teaching skills. Two specific skills worth mentioning include guided thinking and assessing clinical performance.

GUIDING STUDENTS TO THINK

One of the hallmarks of the conceptual approach is helping learners gain higher-order thinking skills. Clinical instructors foster higher-order thinking during clinical experiences by asking thought-provoking questions in a guided thinking process. Guided thinking can also be facilitated through well-designed clinical assignments.

Clinical instructors need to develop skill in questioning students to avoid making them feel as though they are being "grilled," leading to unnecessary stress. There is a tendency for faculty to ask low-level questions where the student merely repeats information they have gained (Phillips et al., 2017). Instead, faculty should encourage students to stretch their thinking beyond obvious answers. The use of open-ended questions that require students to explain their thinking, rationale, and linkage to concepts is desired. Guided instruction in clinical judgment is needed for a student to learn to think like a nurse (Caputi, 2018; Konradi, 2012). Experienced nurses make decisions based on data. They know what information to collect, interpret the meaning of the data, and take appropriate action. When students enter a nursing program, they don't know how nurses solve clinical problems. They need guidance to learn what information is necessary to collect and how to use that information to make decisions that are situation and patient specific. Box 7.9 illustrates a clinical instructor guiding a student through active thinking to facilitate cognitive connections to concepts in clinical practice.

ASSESSING CLINICAL PERFORMANCE

Students require feedback on an ongoing basis; ongoing formative feedback is at the heart of supporting the development of clinical competence. Effective clinical instructors develop skill in accurately assessing performance and providing feedback and coaching in a constructive, nonthreatening way. Competencies, as outcomes statements of concepts, provide clear direction to faculty and students regarding clinical performance expectations. Faculty should avoid premature conclusions based on first impressions—instead, a series of observations are needed over time to allow for improvement and provide a more accurate

---

BOX 7.9 ■ Exemplar: Guiding Students to Think Conceptually

At the beginning of a clinical experience at a geriatric wellness center, Lisa Rubio, a clinical faculty member, has a discussion with Daniel, a junior nursing student, who is working with a patient with anemia. Ms. Rubio asks Daniel about the connection between anemia and the concept Gas Exchange. He states that anemia is associated with decreased hemoglobin, which results in decreased amounts of oxygen available to the body. She then asks Daniel, "What other concepts may be present in a patient with impaired gas exchange?" He replies, "I am not sure, but maybe mobility, nutrition, anxiety, fatigue, and safety."

Ms. Rubio encourages Daniel to collect additional data to investigate the underlying cause of the anemia and the presence of other health conditions to confirm or rule out the presence of these potential interrelated concepts. Understanding the specific pathophysiology of the anemia and other health conditions provides additional information for Daniel to consider for his patient.

Later, as a follow-up to the previous conversation, Ms. Rubio asks Daniel what additional concepts he has considered for his assigned patient. Based on his assessment and chart review, he confirms fatigue as a primary interrelated concept and mentions two other interrelated concepts present: *Care Coordination,* and *Patient Teaching.*

As demonstrated with this example, Daniel reflects on facts and other things he has previously learned to determine patterns. He considers additional information and analyzes this as part of clinical judgment. From a conceptual learning standpoint, this process facilitates cognitive connections, leading to deeper and transferable understandings.

---

assessment. It is particularly important that clinical instructors identify learning needs of students based on an accurate assessment and provide additional instruction where needed. A detailed discussion regarding assessment of student learning is provided in Chapter 8.

Summary

The clinical learning environment represents an epitome for students to apply concepts because this is where nursing practice takes place. Carefully planned CBLAs within the clinical area provide the opportunity for students to expand their conceptual understandings. Concept-based teaching is implemented in all clinical settings, using a variety of teaching strategies to engage students in meaningful conceptual learning. A combination of total patient care and focused clinical activities that address one or more concepts in a patient care area should be developed and incorporated in all clinical courses. These activities must be deliberately planned to ensure students are engaged in learning that is focused on concepts as opposed to a focus on tasks and health conditions. A concept-based curriculum must focus on concepts in all learning environments, including the various clinical settings where nurses practice.

References

Alfayoumi I. The impact of combining concept-based learning and concept-mapping pedagogies on nursing students' clinical reasoning abilities. *Nurse Education Today*. 2019;72:40–46. https://doi.org/10.1016/j.nedt.2018.10.009.

American Association of Colleges of Nursing. *The Essentials: Core Competencies for Professional Nursing Education*. Washington, DC: AACN; 2021. https://www.aacnnursing.org/AACN-Essentials/Download.

Caputi L. *Think Like a Nurse: A Handbook*. Rolling Meadows, IL: Windy City Publishers; 2018.

Daley BJ, Morgan S, Black SB. Concept maps in nursing education: a historical literature review and research directions. *J Nurs Educ*. 2016;55(11):631–639.

Durkin AE, Feinn RS. Traditional and accelerated baccalaureate nursing students' self efficacy for interprofessional learning. *Nurs Educ Perspect*. 2017;38(1):23–28.

Gaberson KB, Oermann M. *Clinical Teaching Strategies in Nursing*. New York, NY: Springer Publishing; 2007.

Giddens J, Brady D. Rescuing nursing education from content saturation: the case for a concept-based curriculum. *J Nurs Educ*. 2007;46(2):65–69.

Gubrud-Howe P, Schoessler M. From random access opportunity to a clinical education curriculum. *J Nurs Educ*. 2008;47(1):3–4.

Hendricks SM, Wangerin V. Concept-based curriculum: changing attitudes and overcoming barriers. *Nurs Educ*. 2017;42(3):138–146.

Institute of Medicine. *Future of Nursing*. Washington, DC: The National Academies Press; 2010.

Interprofessional Education Collaborative. *Interprofessional Education Collaborative: Core Competencies for Interprofessional Collaborative Practice: 2016 Update*. Washington, DC: Interprofessional Education Collaborative; 2016.

Ironside P, McNelis A. *Clinical Education in Prelicensure Nursing Programs: Results From an NLN National Survey*. New York, NY: National League for Nursing; 2010.

Jessee M. Pursing improvement in clinical reasoning: the integrated clinical education theory. *J Nurs Educ*. 2018;57(1):7–13.

Konradi DB. Learning to think like a professional nurse: a critical questions strategy. *J Nurs Educ*. 2012;51:359–360.

Lasater K, Nielsen A. The influence of concept-based learning activities on students' clinical judgment development. *J Nurs Educ*. 2009a;48(8):441–446.

Lasater K, Nielsen A. Reflective journaling for clinical judgment development and evaluation. *J Nurs Educ*. 2009b;48(1):40–44.

Leighton J, Kardong-Edgren S, McNelis AM, et al. Traditional clinical outcomes in prelicensure nursing education: an empty systematic review. *J Nurs Educ*. 2021;60(3):136–142. https://doi.org/10.3928/01484834-20210222-03.

Leighton J, Kardong-Edgren S, McNelis AM, et al. Learning outcomes attributed to prelicensure clinical education in nursing: a systematic review of qualitative research. *Nurse Educ*. 2022;47(1):26–30.

LeFlore JL, Anderson M, Michael JL, et al. Comparison of self-directed learning versus instructor-modeled learning during simulated clinical experience. *Simul Healthc*. 2007;2:170–177.

Lipstein SH, Kellermann AL, Berkowitz B, et al. *Workforce for 21st Century Health and Health Care: A Vital Direction for Health and Health Care*. Washington, DC: National Academies of Medicine; NAM Perspectives. Discussion paper; 2016. https://nam.edu/workforce-for-21st-century-health-and-health-care-a-vital-direction-for-health-and-health-care/.

McNelis AM, Ironside PM, Ebright PR, et al. Learning nursing practice: a multisite, multimethod investigation of clinical education. *J Nurs Regul*. 2014;4(4):30–35.

National Academies of Sciences, Engineering, and Medicine. *The Future of Nursing 2020–2030: Charting a Path to Achieve Health Equity*. Washington, DC: The National Academies Press; 2021.

Nielsen A. Education innovations: concept-based learning activities using the clinical judgment model as a foundation for clinical learning. *J Nurs Educ*. 2009;48:350–354.

Nielsen A. Concept-based learning in clinical experiences: bringing theory to clinical education for deep learning. *J Nurs Educ*. 2016;55(7):365–371.

Nielsen A, Lanciotti K, Garner A, et al. Concept-based learning for capstone clinical experiences in hospital and community settings. *Nurse Educ.* 2021;46(6):381–385. https://doi.org/10.1097/NNE.0000000000000964.

Oermann M, Shellenbarger T, Gaberson K. *Clinical Teaching Strategies in Nursing.* 5th ed. New York, NY: Springer Publishing Company; 2018.

Phillips NM, Duke MM, Weerasuriya R. Questioning skills of clinical facilitators supporting undergraduate nursing students. *J Clin Nurs.* 2017;26(23–24):4344–4352.

Rahnama F, Mardani-Hamooleh M. Iranian nursing students' perceptions regarding use of concept mapping: a concept analysis. *Res Dev Med Educ.* 2017;6(1):45–50. https://doi.org/10.15171/rdme.2017.008.

Repsha CL, Quinn BL, Peters AB. Implementing a concept-based nursing curriculum: a review of the literature. *Teach Learn Nurs.* 2020;15:66–71. https://doi.org/101016/j.teln.2019.09.006.

Senita J. The use of concept maps to evaluate critical thinking in the clinical setting. *Teach Learn Nurs.* 2008;3(1):6–10.

Spector N, Echternacht M. A regulatory model for transitioning newly licensed nurses to practice. *J Nurs Regul.* 2011;1(2):18–25.

Sportsman S, Pleasant T. Concept-based curricula: state of the innovation. *Teach Learn Nurs.* 2017;12:195–200. https://doi.org/10.1016/j.teln.2017.03.001.

Tanner C. From mother duck to mother lode: clinical education for deep learning. *J Nurs Educ.* 2010;49(1):3–4.

Tanner C. Thinking like a nurse: a research-based model of clinical judgment in nursing. *J Nurs Educ.* 2006;45(6):204–211.

Taylor L, Littleton-Keamey M. Concept mapping: a distinctive educational approach to foster critical thinking. *Nur Educator.* 2011;36(2):84–88.

CHAPTER 8

Assessment and Evaluation

Assessment and evaluation are fundamental components of education, thus represent important responsibilities of faculty. Assessment and evaluation occur on many separate yet interrelated levels. On a broad level, nurse educators are accountable for establishing and implementing a process to assess their teaching effectiveness, the courses they teach, curricula, and the overall program. These measures monitor program quality so that improvements can be made to the curriculum and teaching strategies. Through this process, nursing schools can ensure accountability to students, employers, and the general public regarding the quality of the education offered. These activities align with program evaluation (discussed in Chapter 4) and feature many common data-based measures, including licensure pass rates, aggregate assessment of student learning, aggregate course evaluation, and program satisfaction among graduates.

The focus of this chapter is on the assessment and evaluation of student learning with an emphasis on conceptual learning and competency assessment. The terms assessment and evaluation are often used interchangeably—but there is a distinction worth noting. *Assessment* is associated with feedback for improvement in the learning process (while learning is taking place)—whereas *evaluation* tends to be associated with the end point of learning, where a decision or judgment regarding the attainment of learning outcomes occurs. Both assessment and evaluation of student learning are important components of the conceptual approach, and methods must ensure the attainment of learning outcomes and competencies.

The assessment and evaluation of student learning is more challenging than what many think. As established in Chapter 4, learning is a complex cognitive process that results in physiologic changes within the brain—primarily through changes in neural circuitry (Kolb and Whishaw, 2021). These changes cannot be directly measured; thus inferences that learning has occurred are made based on student performance. Many definitions of learning incorporate the notion of change that occurs as a result of learning experiences. Oermann (2015) defines learning as "...an enduring change in behavior, or in the capacity to behave in a given fashion, which results from practice or other forms of experience" (p. 16). Ambrose and colleagues highlight two important points related to learning: (1) "learning is a process, not a product," and (2) "learning is not something done to students, but rather something students themselves do" (Ambrose et al., 2010, p. 3). These definitions and components align closely with the concept-based teaching strategies discussed in Chapters 6 and 7.

Evaluation as a Component of the Educational Process

The educational process involves the components of outcomes, teaching, and evaluation. These components provide the structure for the development of a lesson plan which outlines the lesson outcomes, pre-class preparation, teaching/learning activities, and the planned strategies to assess learning. The development of a lesson plan for concept-based learning activities (CBLAs) was previously discussed in Chapters 6 and 7.

The close interconnected relationship between teaching and learning and between learning and evaluation of that learning should be evident. Teaching involves the skillful sequence of learning events so students can attain the specified learning outcomes and/or competencies. Evaluation of student learning is a process aimed at assessing student learning against established learning outcomes and competencies. These relationships are shown in Fig. 8.1 and discussed further in the following sections.

LEARNING OUTCOMES AND COMPETENCIES

Learning outcomes and competencies are measurable, observable statements that express what is expected of the learner and provide guidelines for instruction. There are two overall types of learning outcomes: program learning outcomes and course learning outcomes.

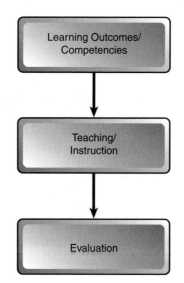

Fig. 8.1 Components of the traditional education process.

- *Program learning outcomes* are broad statements that reflect the characteristics or attributes of the students at the end of the nursing program and the types of behaviors and activities students can engage in by the end of the curriculum. These reflect the nursing program's mission, vision, values, institutional, educational expectations, and national standards related to nursing and health care. Once established, the program learning outcomes and competencies are used to develop the course learning outcomes.
- *Course learning outcomes* reflect expected student learning at the end of a nursing course. These are used to develop the course outline and objectives for each unit, module, or learning session and provide the structure for the assessment and evaluation of student learning within the courses.

TEACHING/INSTRUCTION

The second component is the process of instruction (see Fig. 8.1). A course outline organizes concepts and exemplars and other content into course modules, which are then used to determine teaching methods for each class session. Teaching strategies are designed with the learning outcomes (including learning domain and level), concepts to be learned, and instructional setting (online, classroom, clinical, laboratory) in mind to support students' achievement of the learning outcomes. In other words, teaching and instruction are designed to facilitate learner achievement of the outcomes and competencies.

As discussed in Chapter 5, conceptual learning requires a strong foundation of knowledge on which to build cognitive connections. For this reason, the instruction must include the base knowledge for each concept as well as learning activities that require the application of concepts in a clinical context. Application-level learning activities in didactic and clinical settings provide opportunities for students to develop higher-order thinking and clinical judgment.

EVALUATION

Evaluation represents the third component of the educational process. A broad definition of evaluation is "the process of determining value, worth, or quality" (Bourke and Ihrke, 2016, p. 385). Assessment involves the collection and interpretation of data that lead to a determination regarding student progress and/or achievement of expected outcomes or competencies. Two categories of evaluation include formative and summative.

Formative

Formative evaluation refers to an *assessment* of the learner's progress toward achievement the outcomes or competency and occurs throughout the instructional process. As described by Scheckel, formative evaluation is "conducted while the teaching learning process is unfolding" (Scheckel, 2016, p. 169). From this perspective, formative assessment serves as "diagnostic data" gained through observations and interactions between faculty and students during the instructional process. Lockyer and colleagues (2017) refer to this as "assessment *for* learning" (as opposed to assessment of learning).

The use of audience response systems (otherwise knowns as "clickers") is an example of incorporating formative feedback during a didactic teaching session. Students gain insight regarding their level of understanding, and instructors can easily identify areas that need clarification or further instruction based on aggregate results. This allows for the reinforcement of successful learning and, just as importantly, provides information regarding where further learning is needed. In the clinical setting, formative assessment is commonly done through faculty feedback of a student's clinical performance based on an evaluation tool—thus providing an opportunity for improvement. Considering the important role of assessment as part of the learning process, it is shown in Fig. 8.2 as a feedback loop within the instructional process.

Summative

Summative evaluation occurs at the endpoint of the educational process and is used to determine if the learner has met the achieved outcomes and competencies; these are critical measures used at specified points in time to determine course grades and/or academic progression. Lockyer and colleagues (2017) refer to this as an "assessment *of* learning."

The lesson plan should indicate the mechanism for assessment—examinations, clinical evaluation tools, formal papers, and student presentations as examples. Summative evaluation strategies align with program and course learning objectives because all curricular components are linked. Methods used to evaluate the achievement of learning outcomes are varied and must align with the appropriate domain and level of the learning outcomes.

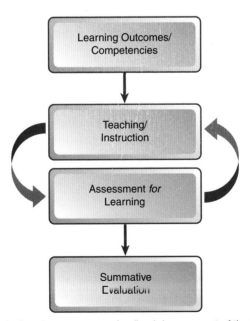

Fig. 8.2 Assessment for learning serves as a feedback loop as part of the instructional process.

Developing an Assessment and Evaluation Strategy

A variety of strategies should be used to assess and evaluate student learning because multiple opportunities for assessment using a variety of strategies provide a more complete and accurate representation of the student's abilities. Faculty should consider several factors when making decisions regarding an assessment or evaluation strategy, including:

- *purpose* or goal of the assessment or evaluation;
- *domain* of learning reflected by the learning outcome;
- instructional *setting* where the assessment or evaluation will take place;
- *process* required to conduct the assessment.
- *measurement* and tools used to conduct the assessment or evaluation

PURPOSE/GOAL

The preceding discussion regarding formative assessment and summative evaluation flows nicely into a conversation regarding the purpose or goal of the evaluation. If the purpose or goal of the assessment is to provide feedback to students for improvement, then a formative approach is selected. Alternatively, if the primary goal is to form a definitive decision about the learning, then a summative evaluation strategy is used, with a plan regarding the value or weight the evaluation element carries toward the final course grade or decision point.

LEARNING DOMAINS

Another factor to consider in the selection of the assessment or evaluation strategy is the domain of learning reflected in the learning outcomes. Learning outcomes reflect one of three learning domains based on Bloom's taxonomy (cognitive, psychomotor, and affective), each with an associated hierarchy of complexity (Anderson and Krathwohl, 2001; Bloom, 1956). The cognitive domain relates to knowledge, knowledge acquisition, and intellectual capacity and thus is often evaluated through testing, writing, and portfolios. The psychomotor domain deals with skill development associated with the execution of clinically based interventions and the use of technology. Common strategies include simulation, clinical laboratory skills testing, and clinical performance assessment. The affective domain, which is often considered the hardest to measure, involves the development of one's values, beliefs, and attitudes in the context of professional nursing care. Most assessment strategies can be adapted for or have a component of the strategy address this domain. (See Chapter 6 for additional information about these domains and hierarchies.) Box 8.1 presents common assessment and evaluation strategies and applicable learning domains represented.

INSTRUCTIONAL SETTING

The instructional setting represents another factor to consider as assessment and evaluation strategies are determined; many can be used in any setting. As an

> **BOX 8.1 ■ Common Assignments and Strategies to Evaluate Student Learning and Applicable Domains**
>
> - Examination/Tests (Cognitive)
> - Oral Questioning (Cognitive, Affective)
> - Written Paper (multiple variations) (Cognitive, Affective)
> - Reflective Writing (Cognitive, Affective)
> - Portfolio (Cognitive, Affective, Psychomotor)
> - Case Study (Cognitive, Affective)
> - Presentations (Cognitive, Affective)
> - Role Play (Cognitive, Affective, Psychomotor)
> - Concept Map (Cognitive, Affective)
> - Observation/Clinical Performance (Cognitive, Affective, Psychomotor)
> - Simulation (Cognitive, Affective, Psychomotor)

example, written papers are assigned in clinical and classroom settings, but it is the context of the assignment that makes the evaluation process unique. That said, some settings naturally lend themselves to certain assessment and evaluation approaches—such as a written examination in a didactic course. However, the use of technologies (such as online examinations) has made the setting less important. Assessment of clinical performance is conducted in a clinical setting—including a clinical laboratory, simulated clinical environment, or within a patient care area. Increasingly outcomes of clinical learning are expressed in the form of clinical competencies to be demonstrated; thus, an appropriate setting to observe clinical performance is necessary.

PROCESS

The process for assessment and evaluation represents a myriad of variables for consideration. The amount of time needed, special equipment or technologies needed, and the assessment or evaluation tools used (i.e., examinations, rubrics, clinical evaluation documents) are just a few examples. If technologies are used in the assessment or evaluation process, students and evaluators must be familiar with the technology being used. Observation is the most common strategy for evaluating clinical performance (Oermann et al., 2009); thus, an equitable and consistent process depends on using valid and reliable tools. This is particularly important when multiple faculty are involved in the evaluation process.

MEASUREMENT

Measurement, as a component of assessment and evaluation, refers to the assignment of a value (such as a number) to demonstrate "how much" or "to what degree" a student demonstrates performance or achievement but does not represent a judgment of quality. Scores on examinations, papers, and other measurement methods serve only as a reference point on an expected standard. Measurement is useful as an indirect measure of learning and for the purposes of assigning a grade on an assignment, test, or course grade. A single measurement does not typically provide an indication of attainment of all learning outcomes. The interpretation of measurement scores occurs through norm-referenced and criterion-referenced approaches.

Norm Referenced and Criterion-Referenced Approaches

In a *norm-referenced approach*, an individual student's score is compared to others (in the class, clinical, or another relevant group for referencing) from the standpoint of ranking within the class. In other words, the measure is affected by the performance of others in the class. The limitation to norm referencing is that it does not actually confirm what a student has learned or can do—it only measures the student in comparison to others. In contrast to the norm-referenced approach, a *criterion-referenced approach* is based on a preset standard or criteria. The interpretation includes a measure of what the student can do, a percentage of correct or incorrect answers, and a determination of the attainment of the specified standard. The standards are made explicit to faculty and students so there is clarity regarding what is expected. Thus, student performance reflects what the student learned or did—and is not impacted by the performance of others within the class. Most evaluation in nursing education follows a criterion-referenced approach.

Assessment and Evaluation Tools

A fair and reliable assessment or evaluation process requires the use of tools that measure what is intended and in a consistent way among all faculty involved in the process. Although it is impossible to create a "perfect" tool that is completely free of subjectivity and bias, there are measures one can take to reduce such variability. Tools should be developed that are criterion-referenced and align with intended learning outcomes and/or competencies; furthermore, these should be clear and relatively easy to use.

Rating scales such as a grading rubric provide greater latitude for evaluation. The scale incorporates a list of descriptors reflecting the level of performance or achievement and a scale to rate the performance for each. A rubric can be developed to evaluate nearly any type of assignment and are particularly useful for the assessment or evaluation of written assignments and observational evaluation (often as a clinical evaluation tool). Rubrics or rating scales should be included as part of the assignment or evaluation strategy design.

Checklists are another type of tool often used in a clinical setting and provide a recording of the completion of steps or things accomplished. Many checklists are used in a laboratory setting as part of skills assessments and represent a dichotomous variable for each step: satisfactory or unsatisfactory performance; pass/fail; did/not did. Students may find these helpful in preparation for skills evaluation, but checklists don't necessarily represent an assessment of the quality of performance.

Progress notes (also known as anecdotal notes) are written descriptions of what is observed and thus are useful for observational evaluation. Program notes can take on a structured format to connect behaviors to learning objectives. These are particularly helpful in documenting patterns of behavior and/or progress over time and are useful for formative evaluation.

Assessment and Evaluation in the Context of the Conceptual Approach

The principles of assessment and evaluation presented in the preceding sections are applicable in any education setting and within every discipline. Thus, these principles also form the foundation for the assessment of conceptual learning. The *process* of assessment or evaluation of student learning is the same, but the hallmark of evaluation of learning in the conceptual approach is the *focus* of the process—in other words, what is assessed and how. Methods must ensure assessment of learning outcomes and competencies as they relate to the conceptual, organizational structure for content delivery. This requires careful consideration of conceptual learning outcomes and competencies from a framework that supports assessment in the context of healthcare. Student performance should be clearly linked to the application of the concept used in the curriculum. An example showing all elements from program learning outcomes through evaluation for the concept of *Collaboration* is shown in Box 8.2.

Conceptual learning involves building cognitive connections through the application of concepts in multiple contexts and the transferability of information previously learned to new situations. Thus, a central aspect of evaluating student learning is the students' ability to transfer learning about a concept from one situation to another. *Can the students use what they have learned in a new*

BOX 8.2 ■ Evaluation of *Collaboration* From Program Outcome to Class Evaluation

Program Learning Outcome
- Participate in collaboration and teamwork with members of the interprofessional team, the patient, and the patient's support persons.

Leadership Course Learning Outcome
- Compare and contrast techniques used to develop collaborative relationships with members of the interprofessional team, the patient, and the patient's support persons when caring for patients with complex, high-acuity conditions.

Class/Lesson Objective
- Analyze interprofessional communication and collaboration skills used to deliver safe, evidence-based, patient-centered care.

Classroom Teaching Methods
- Concept presentation, Collaboration
- Case study review
- Small group discussion

Evaluation
- Classroom test items, in-class assignments, clinical evaluation tool

situation? Just as a child who learns multiplication tables must be able to determine when to use that math skill, so it is with the learning of concepts. Students who learn about a concept must be able to discern when knowledge of that concept should be used in a particular context as appropriate for safe patient care (Benner et al., 2010). These are essential skills necessary as a foundation for clinical judgment. Thus, assessment methods in a concept-based curriculum should provide opportunities for students to demonstrate they are able to apply their learning to new situations.

MISCONCEPTIONS AND CLARIFICATIONS

Misconception: The conceptual approach requires completely different strategies to assess and evaluate student learning.

Clarification: Faculty will continue to use many of the same strategies but with a different focus. The focus of evaluation for the conceptual approach is the students' ability to transfer conceptual information from one situation to another. A focus on the application of an in-depth knowledge of concepts is at the heart of evaluation of student learning.

COMMON ASSESSMENT AND EVALUATION METHODS

Methods used to evaluate student achievement of learning outcomes should link to the concepts, so the evaluation of conceptual learning is clearly delineated. As mentioned previously, assessment and evaluation should occur over multiple points of time using a wide variety of valid and reliable tools. Furthermore, the assessment and evaluation approach should demonstrate a connection to a course learning outcome that relates to the concept-based curriculum. Examples of four common evaluation strategies are presented in the sections that follow showing how these are used to assess conceptual learning.

Classroom Examinations

One method for evaluating student achievement of course learning outcomes is a written examination. Faculty use a test blueprint that directly links a test item to the lesson objective, which is linked to the course learning outcome. If students are able to answer the test items linked to the lesson objective and the test items are determined to be reliable on the basis of item analysis, faculty can determine whether students are achieving the course learning outcome related to a given concept. Written examinations evaluate learning associated with concepts taught during the classroom sessions, as well as the exemplars used for concept application. For example, with regard to the *lesson objective* example in Box 8.2, a test item focused on the concept of *Collaboration* may have the following stem:

Present a patient situation. Then ask: Which collaborative action will the nurse take?

This question is focused on a patient situation while asking a question about the concept of *Collaboration*. An alternate approach to evaluating students' understanding of *Collaboration* is to present the question in the following way:

Present a patient situation. Then ask: Which action will the nurse take?

The actions listed in the options reflect a number of different alternatives, one of which represents a *collaborative* behavior without using the word "collaboration." This type of question evaluates the students' understanding of when to apply *Collaboration* to a situation.

The cognitive level of questions should match the course learning outcomes, and the questions should determine the understanding of concepts via application and analysis of the concepts at a level appropriate to the course. For example, a simple application question may be:

Present a patient situation. Then ask: Which concepts will the nurse further investigate?

The stem of this question does not ask about a specific concept; rather, students must draw from the patient situation to determine concepts that need further investigation.

Questions directed at the application of concepts related to exemplars are also included in examinations. An example of a question related to the concept of *Pain* experienced by a patient during the postoperative period may be:

The nurse assesses a patient 2 days after open abdominal surgery. The patient reports diffuse abdominal discomfort. The nurse notes the absence of bowel sounds, distention, and lack of flatus. The nurse should implement which intervention?

It is important to determine not only the concept but the cognitive level of the learning outcome and competency, then write the test item to match both. Table 8.1 provides examples of test items focused on the concept of *Anxiety*. Note these represent three versions of the test item, one written at the knowledge level, one at the comprehension level, and one at the application level.

All the aforementioned questions represent a focus on concepts applied to patient situations. By using a test blueprint, each question can be linked to a course learning outcome that represents specific concepts. Faculty can analyze test results to determine which questions were or were not effective at measuring student learning. This analysis should look at the individual student to provide individual remediation for the student. However, the analysis should also focus on how the students answered each question as a group. With this information, the faculty determines if remediation or reteaching of the concept is needed for the class as a whole (or considers the possibility that the test question was flawed). This analysis provides information about student achievement of

TABLE 8.1 ■ **Test Items Focused on the Concept of *Anxiety* at Three Cognitive Levels**

Cognitive Level	Test Item
Knowledge (Remembering)	A 44-year-old patient is admitted to the outpatient surgical center for a minor surgical procedure. Which assessment data indicates the patient may be experiencing anxiety? 1. Lab results indicate fasting blood glucose of 96. 2. Heart rate 110; blood pressure 130/85 3. Respiratory rate of 12 4. Quiet tone of voice
Comprehension (Understanding)	A 44-year-old patient is admitted to the outpatient surgical center for a minor surgical procedure. Which statement by the patient prompts the nurse to further investigate the presence of anxiety? 1. My girlfriend will be here soon and would like to be with me when she arrives. 2. How many patients are having surgery today? 3. How long will I be here after the surgery? 4. My friend had this same surgery and ended up in the ICU.
Application (Applying)	A 44-year-old patient is admitted to the outpatient surgical center for a minor surgical procedure. The patient's vitals are: BP: 140/90, P: 90, T: 98.4; R: 22. The patient tells the nurse this is his first experience with surgery. What is the nurse's first action? 1. Check the chart for surgical consent. 2. Discuss postoperative care of the incision. 3. Assess the patient's ability to walk to the bathroom for a urine specimen. 4. Ask if he has specific concerns he would like to address at this time.

specific learning outcomes and the concepts related to those learning outcomes. This information is necessary to guide the faculty's actions to improve the course based on poor performance related to identified learning outcomes.

Written Assignments

Written assignments are a commonly used evaluation method in nursing education that can be used in any learning environment. Written assignments can take on a variety of formats (such as formal research-based papers, short written assignments, reflective writing, care plans, portfolios, and case-based reports, to name a few), thus can be used to evaluate cognitive and/or affective domains of learning. Formal papers provide opportunities for students to demonstrate their knowledge of one or more concepts and their ability to apply higher-level thinking. Faculty should include guidelines for the written assignment so that students are clear about the expectations and how the paper will be evaluated.

As an example, from the context of conceptual learning, the concept of *Collaboration* will again be used as an exemplar. The course learning outcome presented earlier can be used for this purpose:

Compare and contrast techniques used to develop collaborative relationships with members of the interprofessional team, the patient, and the patient's support persons when caring for patients with complex, high-acuity conditions.

The purpose of this written assignment (Box 8.3) is for the student to compare and contrast collaboration among the interprofessional team members in two health care settings. A grading rubric used to evaluate student performance on the assignment is presented in Table 8.2. An assignment like this would be appropriate for a course at the upper level because it requires students to have had clinical experiences in several different agencies or on several different units in one health care agency.

Clinical Performance

Several learning strategies are used in the clinical environment and thus a number of assignments and tools are used to assess and evaluate clinical performance. These tools are used to assess progress or confirm the achievement of competencies as they relate to performance in the clinical environment. In a concept-based curriculum, the course learning outcomes represent important nursing concepts. Thus, the assessment incorporates the application of the concepts within the clinical environment.

Continuing with the example of *Collaboration*, a clinical rubric is developed to evaluate this concept. The course learning outcome presented earlier can be used for this purpose: *Compare and contrast techniques used to develop collaborative*

BOX 8.3 ■ Sample Written Assignment for the Concept of Collaboration

Goal of Assignment: Write a paper comparing and contrasting the concept of *Collaboration* among members of the health care team in two health care settings.

1. Using the following three attributes of the concept of *Collaboration*, discuss how collaboration among the members of the health care team in each of the settings was similar and how it was different.
   - Roles and responsibilities
   - Communication
   - Teams and teamwork
2. For the concept of *Collaboration*, choose two interrelated concepts. Discuss how they were exemplified in each of the settings. Discuss how the settings were the same and different.
3. Draw conclusions about the collaboration you experienced in each of the health care settings. Discuss and explain why you would choose one setting over the other. Provide rationales for your selection.

TABLE 8.2 ■ Sample Grading Rubric

Grading Rubric	Excellent: 3 Points	Good: 2 Points	Fair: 1 Point	Unacceptable: 0 Points
1. Using three attributes of the concept of *Collaboration*, discuss how collaboration among the members of the health care team in each of the settings was similar and how it was different.	Discussion is complete, explicit, and focused.	Discussion is complete and clearly written, with minor areas incomplete.	Discussion is generally complete but lacks significant information.	Discussion is scant, superficial, and lacking in detail.
2. For the concept of *Collaboration*, choose two interrelated concepts, discuss how they were exemplified in each of the settings, and discuss how the settings were the same and different.	Discussion is complete, explicit, and focused.	Discussion is complete and clearly written, with minor areas incomplete.	Discussion is generally complete but lacks significant information.	Discussion is scant, superficial, and lacking in detail.
3. Draw conclusions about the collaboration you experienced in each of the health care settings; discuss and explain why you would choose one setting over the other, providing rationales for your selection.	Discussion is complete, explicit, and focused.	Discussion is complete and clearly written, with minor areas incomplete.	Discussion is generally complete but lacks significant information.	Discussion is scant, superficial, and lacking in detail.

relationships with members of the interprofessional team, the patient, and the patient's support persons when caring for patients with complex, high-acuity conditions.

Students engage in clinical learning activities that demonstrate their ability to analyze *Collaboration* among health care team members. Box 8.4 presents an example of a concept-based learning activity (CBLA) featuring collaboration that

---

BOX 8.4 ■ CBLA: Collaboration and Conflict Resolution

1. Interview a nurse and one other healthcare professional to describe an area of conflict in the clinical area they have experienced among other healthcare professionals and how the conflict was resolved.
2. Observe the interactions of health care professionals. What conflicts did you observe? How were they handled or not handled?
3. What conflict resolution principles were evident in the situations described to you by the nurse and health care professional and those you observed on the unit? How would you approach these conflicts? Explain your approach incorporating conflict resolution principles.

CBLA, *Concept-based learning activity.*

TABLE 8.3 ■ Grading Rubric for Conflict Resolution Clinical Activity

Performance Criteria	Satisfactory: 2 Points	Needs Improvement: 1 Point	Unsatisfactory: 0 Point
Conflicts identified in the unit	Clearly describes conflicts in the unit	Descriptions of conflicts in the unit are vague and unclear.	Unable to describe any conflicts in the unit
Explanation of how to resolve a conflict	Clearly and accurately explains how to handle the conflict	Explanation of handling the conflict is scant and not well substantiated.	Unable to explain how to handle the conflict

Copyright Linda Caputi, Inc. Used with permission.

---

directs students to analyze the activities and behaviors of the interprofessional team for the purpose of learning to deal with conflict, an important communication skill used when engaging in a collaborative relationship. A grading rubric (Table 8.3) increases objectivity and consistency in the assessment or evaluation process.

The assessment of a learning activity such as this can be used as a measure of individual student performance or evidence of learning for a group of students. To determine whether the class as a group is meeting expected outcomes on an assignment, an aggregate score is calculated among all students completing the assignment and evaluated against a predetermined metric. For example, if the predetermined metric is that 90% of the class achieves "satisfactory," then the aggregate mean score would be 1.8 or higher. Alternatively, the faculty can determine the total number of students achieving "satisfactory" divided by the total number of students in the class to determine whether the 90% metric is achieved. The aggregate score provides information about the level of learning for the class, indicating areas of strength and weakness of the assignment, the course, or the curriculum. Any indication of poor performance prompts faculty to determine changes that might be made to enhance the students' learning of the concept of *Collaboration*.

Concept Maps

Concept maps are common assignments in didactic or clinical learning environments. A concept map is a graphic representation of key concepts related to a patient and related nursing care (Oermann et al., 2018) and serves as a useful method for formative assessment. The student organizes and integrates information about their patient as well as information from their readings to show key connections between and among concepts. There is no one format for a concept map; these can be structured or left to the creativity of the student. Initially, students may benefit from a structured approach by using a concept map template (a simple example is shown in Fig. 8.3). In the example shown, students place specified information about the patient in the center of the map and priority concepts as determined by the student. Over time, with deeper conceptual understanding and experience using concept maps, students may benefit from creating their own unique concept map designs.

In the clinical environment, the concept map is updated and refined as the student engages in clinical care with the patient—such as performing assessments, making decisions, and deciding on interventions. By showing the integration of concepts, clinical care activities, and linkages between and among

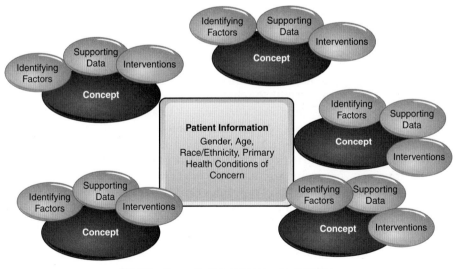

Fig. 8.3 Example of a concept map template.

the concepts, it provides faculty with a wealth of knowledge about the students' understanding of concepts and linkages among interrelated concepts and insights into how the student is thinking. The map is a useful way for faculty to provide feedback during the clinical experience, thus helping students refine their thinking throughout the clinical experience. A concept map may also be used in the classroom or clinical setting as a summative evaluation based on an actual patient or a case-based learning activity. When the intent is for a summative assessment, a grading rubric should be used to establish a criterion-referenced approach to assigning a grade.

Assessment of Clinical Competence

A significant shift toward competency-based assessment is underway in health sciences education—including nursing. Competency-based assessment involves an intentional assessment of clinical performance. The increased emphasis on competencies in health sciences education has emerged, partly due to a call for greater accountability of graduates to have a consistent set of core knowledge and skills (Lucey, 2018). The concern is well illustrated by researchers who reported a continued decline in the initial preparedness of new nursing graduates (Kavanagh and Sharpnack, 2021).

As discussed in Chapter 2, competencies are closely tied to concepts; their relationship is best described as complementary. The concept (or domain) represents an overarching idea or collection of information representing important disciplinary knowledge, whereas a competency is an outcome statement that stipulates the behaviors and performance expectations related to the concept in clinical practice. Put another way, "whereas concepts represent the structural organization of knowledge to be learned, competencies provide the structure and process for performance and assessment" (Giddens, 2020, p. 124).

MODEL FOR COMPETENCY ASSESSMENT

The medicine discipline has been the front runner of competency-based education and, thus, has grappled with the challenges of competency assessment. Over three decades ago, Miller proposed a framework to assess competence, emphasizing that no single strategy can provide all information needed required to determine a student's competence (Miller, 1990). Today, this framework remains relevant as a useful way to explain the assessment of competencies within a conceptual approach. According to Miller, the evaluation process should confirm that the learner has acquired new knowledge (knows what is required for clinical practice), knows how to use the knowledge in a clinical context, and then shows how that information is applied. The evaluation of learning includes both cognitive assessment and the evaluation of clinical performance. Ideally, such an approach can predict how a graduate will do once they are in clinical practice.

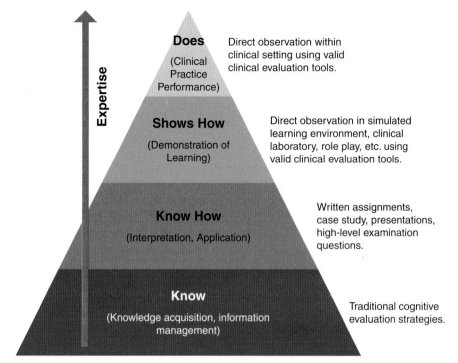

Fig. 8.4 Modified Miller's framework for competency assessment. (Adapted from Miller GE. The assessment of clinical skills/competence/performance. *Acad Med*. 1990;65(9):S63–S67.)

An adaptation of Miller's framework is shown in Fig. 8.4. Students first have a solid conceptual understanding as a foundation representing cognitive assessments often conducted in a didactic course setting. Clinical performance assessment occurs in a clinical context, representing a behavioral assessment whereby the student demonstrates what they can do. Competencies are not to be confused with clinical checklists or tasks. Although a check list might be used as one component of competency assessment, competencies require an *integration* of multiple components including knowledge, skills, attitudes, and values (which mirror the learning domains previously discussed). There must be multiple, appropriate clinical experiences allowing students sufficient opportunities to achieve the stated competencies. Furthermore, competencies are not to be confused with course learning outcomes. When competencies are written at a programmatic level, assessment and evaluation of competencies occur across the program; gains in conceptual understandings and experience lead to greater expertise over time.

Another important consideration regarding competency assessment is that the process is not a linear approach, particularly at the upper end of Miller's framework. In other words, it would be unusual to assess a single competency in isolation of others because competencies are demonstrated in the context of care delivery and clinical performance. Thus, an assessment will typically provide data for multiple competencies during a clinical encounter.

MISCONCEPTIONS AND CLARIFICATIONS

Misconception: A learning outcome is the same thing as a competency.	**Clarification:** There are many similarities between learning outcomes and competencies. Both are outcome statements regarding what is expected of the learner as a result of learning. However, an important distinction exists. A learning outcome is written in alignment with one learning domain (cognitive, psychomotor, or affective). A competency describes a performance expectation that requires an **integration** of knowledge, skills, and values.

FACULTY ROLE IN COMPETENCY ASSESSMENT

A known challenge associated with observational assessment is the introduction of the personal values, beliefs, and biases introduced by evaluators—in other words, subjectivity can lead to inconsistent evaluation of performance. Agreement and shared understanding among faculty regarding the performance standard are essential. As an example, a competency statement for the concept of Collaboration might be:

Establish appropriate relationships with members of the health care team.

Without clarity, this competency may hold different meanings for different faculty, or one faculty member may be looking for something different than another faculty. For this reason, rigorous criterion-based methods are needed to evaluate clinical performance. The use of "sub-competencies" is one way to further articulate what is expected for competency achievement, particularly if evaluating the same competency with different levels of learners. One way to think about the value of a sub-competency is that they "paint a picture of how the competency is achieved..." (American Association of Colleges of Nursing, 2021, p. 15), thus, representing a collection of behaviors that describe the achievement of the parent competency.

Competency-based assessment represents a shift in nursing education because it places a much greater emphasis on formative assessment in recognition that competency development is a process that occurs over time. From this perspective, the instructor directly observes the student and provides just-in-time clinical coaching, thereby giving the student an opportunity to improve their performance. An analogy that may make this approach clearer is the process of learning to play a musical instrument.

A novice musician gains a base knowledge of the meaning of symbols that represent notes and also a base understanding how to create the corresponding notes on the instrument. A music teacher coaches the student on everything from how to use the instrument, to learning how to read and interpret the music with a multitude of variations in notes (pitch and duration) and rhythm so that the music can be played. Over time, the novice gains greater knowledge, skill, and appreciation for the music as ongoing feedback is provided.

Imagine making a judgment about the competence and skill of a musician solely based on a cognitive test on notes. Alternatively, imagine expecting a novice to practice for an extended period without the benefit of feedback or coaching and then making a final judgment on their skill based on a single performance. With this analogy in mind, the role of the nursing faculty member becomes clearer as it relates to competency-based assessment.

As stated by Virk and colleagues, assessment is "a part and parcel of instruction rather than being an appendage of the process" (Virk et al., 2020, p. 203), a point well reflected previously in Fig. 8.3. For faculty, coaching has been identified as the skill most commonly described as a core component of competency-based assessment (Holmboe et al., 2011; Hawkins et al., 2015; Sirianni et al., 2020; Walsh et al., 2018). A comprehensive assessment plan with a variety of valid and reliable assessment tools are needed (particularly considering multiple faculty are involved with assessments) as well as a tracking matrix to document progression over time. Oermann encourages us to think about a "program of assessment" over time as opposed to strictly thinking about evaluating a student in a course or simulation (Oermann, 2022). Thus, an evaluation mindset requires faculty training in competency assessment. A challenge in implementing competency-based evaluation noted in the medical literature is a lack of competency assessment tools and gaps in assessment skills among faculty (Shorey et al., 2019; Sirianni et al., 2020). Thus, nurse educators should expect that the shift to competency-based assessment will require faculty training in competency assessment.

Summary

Evaluation of conceptual learning follows standard principles of evaluation, but with an emphasis on conceptual understanding in the context of clinical practice. The evaluation process should incorporate many strategies and over time, not only to give students an opportunity to improve, based on feedback, but also to document attainment of the learning outcomes and competency. As competency-based education becomes more prominent in health sciences education, nursing education is well poised to incorporate this approach. Because competencies are outcome statements associated with concepts, competency-based evaluation aligns closely with the concept-based approach. With the recent adoption of the AACN *Essentials* (2021), nursing faculty can expect to see conceptual approaches and competency evaluation to become more prominent. This will require a change in how many schools have approached evaluation and will require adopting an "evaluation mindset" and faculty training for robust evaluation of conceptual learning and competence.

References

American Association of Colleges of Nursing. *The Essentials: Core Competencies for Professional Nursing Education.* Washington, DC: American Association of College of Nursing; 2021. Retrieve from: https://www.aacnnursing.org/AACN-Essentials/Download.

Ambrose SA, Bridges MW, DiPietro M, et al. *How Learning Works.* San Francisco, CA: Jossey-Bass; 2010.

Anderson LW, Krathwohl DR. *A Taxonomy for Learning, Teaching, and Assessing: A Revision of Blooms' Taxonomy of Educational Objectives.* New York, NY: Longman; 2001.

Benner P, Sutphen M, Leonard V, et al. *Educating Nurses: A Call for Radical Transformation.* Stanford, CA: Jossey-Bass; 2010.

Bloom BS. *Taxonomy of Educational Objectives.* New York: Longman; 1956.

Bourke MP, Ihrke BA. Introduction to the evaluation process. In: Billings DM, Halstead JA, eds. *Teaching in Nursing: A Guide for Faculty.* 5th ed. St. Louis, MO: Elsevier; 2016.

Giddens J. Demystifying concept-based and competency-based approaches. *J Nurs Educ.* 2020;59(3): 123–124.

Hawkins RE, Welcher CM, Holmboe ES, et al. Implementation of a competency-based medical education: are we addressing the concerns and challenges? *Med Educ.* 2015;49(11):1086–1102.

Holmboe ES, Ward DS, Reznick RJ, et al. Faculty development in assessment: the missing link in competency-based medical education. *Acad Med.* 2011;86(4):460–467.

Kavanagh JM, Sharpnack PA. Crisis in competency: a defining moment in nursing education. *Online J Issues Nurs.* 2021;26(1).

Kolb B, Whishaw IQ. *Fundamentals of Human Neuropsychology.* 8th ed. New York, NY: Worth Publishers; 2021.

Lockyer J, Carraccio C, Chan MK, et al. Core principles of assessment in competency-based medical education. *Med Teach.* 2017;39(6):609–616.

Lucey CR. Achieving competency-based time variable health professions education. In: *Proceedings of a Conference Sponsored by Josiah Macy Jr. Foundation in June 2017.* New York, NY: Josiah Macy Jr. Foundation; 2018.

Miller GE. The assessment of clinical skills/competence/performance. *Acad Med.* 1990;65(9). September Supplement:S63–S67.

Oermann MH. *Teaching in Nursing and Role of the Educator.* New York, NY: Springer; 2015.

Oermann MH. Some principles to guide assessment of competencies. *Nurse Educ.* 2022;47(1):1.

Oermann MH, Shellenbarger T, Gaberson KB. *Clinical Teaching Strategies in Nursing.* 5th ed. New York, NY: Springer; 2018.

Oermann MH, Yarbrough SS, Ard N, et al. Clinical evaluation and grading practices in schools of nursing: national survey findings part II. *Nurs Educ Perspect.* 2009;30:274–279.

Scheckel M. Designing courses and learning experiences. In: Billings DM, Halstead JA, eds. *Teaching in Nursing: A Guide for Faculty.* 5th ed. St. Louis, MO: Elsevier; 2016.

Shorey S, Lau TC, Lau ST, et al. Entrustable professional activities in health care education: a scoping review. *Med Educ.* 2019;53:766–777.

Sirianni G, Takahashi SG, Meyers J. Taking stock of what is known about faculty development in competency-based medical education: a scoping review paper. *Med Teach.* 2020;42(8):909–915.

Virk A, Joshi A, Mahajan R, et al. The power of subjectivity in competency-based assessment. *J Postgrad Med.* 2020;66(4):200–205.

Walsh A, Koppula S, Antao V, et al. Preparing teachers for competency-based medical education: fundamental etching activities. *Med Teach.* 2018;40(1):80–85.

CHAPTER 9

Advancing the Conceptual Approach in Nursing

Throughout this book, the conceptual approach is presented to help nurse educators successfully implement a concept-based curriculum, concept-based instruction, and evaluation of conceptual learning. Effective and sustained implementation requires a commitment from the faculty, individually and collectively, to continually develop expertise in this area. This chapter presents an overview of the nursing literature to date and areas for further inquiry, considerations for the professional development of nursing faculty with proposed competencies, and the future potential for the conceptual approach to be adopted across health-sciences education.

What Do We Know About Conceptual Approach From the Nursing Literature?

Although conceptual learning has been well represented in the education literature for decades, the conceptual approach has only recently become prevalent in nursing literature. The primary areas of literature include articles that describe the conceptual approach movement, articles describing concept-based curriculum development and implementation, articles describing outcomes, and articles describing teaching strategies to facilitate conceptual learning.

THE CONCEPTUAL APPROACH MOVEMENT

The current conceptual approach movement in nursing began in the mid-2000s. Evidence of the rise in interest and adoption of the conceptual approach is demonstrated through the number of articles published in the nursing literature. Using search terms "concept-based" and "nursing education," a search in the CINAHL database between 1990 and 2000 produced one published article. Between 2000 and 2010, the number grew by 12 published articles; between 2010 and 2022, an additional 67 articles were published in the nursing literature. The extent of this movement is also reflected by the recent emergence of international articles (published in English) within the nursing literature, including Australia, Africa, China, Hong Kong, Iran, Jordan, New Zealand, Malaysia, and Taiwan, and the emergence of the conceptual approach in graduate nursing education.

Not surprisingly, some of the first articles that appear in the nursing literature describe the conceptual approach phenomenon. One of the earliest articles proposed the conceptual approach as a way to address increasing concerns regarding excessive content in nursing curricula (Giddens and Brady, 2007). Specifically, the authors described how a concept-based curriculum and conceptual teaching differed from a traditional nursing curriculum and teaching practices and how this approach could lead to a reduction in curriculum content. Brandon and All (2010) presented a theoretical basis for the conceptual approach through the lens of constructivism learning theory and student-centered learning. The authors postulated that a constructivist approach using concepts and active teaching promotes critical thinking skills and builds confidence among students. More recently, several articles have appeared in publications targeting practicing registered nurses to inform their readers about trends in nursing education that affect the preparation of new nurses entering practice (Allen, 2013; Goodman, 2014; Trossman, 2015).

CONCEPT-BASED CURRICULUM DEVELOPMENT AND IMPLEMENTATION

Many articles published to date in the nursing literature describe concept-based curricula. Not surprisingly, these articles focus predominantly on the description of the curriculum design (Giddens et al., 2008; Hollinshead and Stirling, 2014; Patterson et al., 2016; Popoola, 2012) or the process of curriculum development and implementation (Brady et al., 2008; Giddens et al., 2012; Hendricks and Wangerin, 2017; Hollinshead and Stirling, 2014; McGrath, 2015; Patterson et al., 2016; Popoola, 2012; Pyatt, 2021). As part of curriculum development, several articles discussed methods to select concepts and concept development for the curriculum (Brussow et al., 2019; Christmasles et al., 2019; Crookes et al., 2020; Giddens et al., 2012; Herrington and Schneidereith, 2017). Repsha et al. (2020) conducted a review of the literature regarding the implementation a concept-based curriculum in nursing and reported that several methods were used for development and design. Two articles describe a specific curriculum framework or model as part of the curriculum design process (Hollinshead and Stirling, 2014; Popoola, 2012). The conceptual approach was also reported as the foundation for a statewide academic progression model (Giddens et al., 2015) and facilitates registered nurse progression to the baccalaureate degree (Repsha et al., 2020).

As multiple schools adopted the conceptual approach, a number of studies were conducted to learn about faculty perceptions and experiences (Sportsman and Pleasant, 2017; Wilhelm et al., 2020; Zhu et al., 2022). Common themes include challenges associated with faculty making the adjustment to a new approach and addressing concerns regarding competing demands in curriculum development. The need for faculty development and administrative support was also noted consistently. Gaining full commitment among faculty to adopt concept-based teaching strategies is a common barrier to success (Giddens, 2016). Sportsman and Pleasant (2017) proposed an implementation checklist for faculty considering adopting a concept-based curriculum.

CONCEPT-BASED CURRICULUM OUTCOMES

In general, curriculum evaluation is a topic with limited visibility in the nursing literature. Even less is written on the process of evaluating a concept-based curriculum or published program metrics. Common metrics for curriculum and program evaluation include first-time NLCEX-RN pass rates, standardized test measurements, time to graduation, graduation rates, and satisfaction (student, employer, and/or alumni).

Five published articles reported on NCLEX pass rates as a curriculum outcome after the adoption of a concept-based curriculum; four of these reported no change to the NCLEX pass rates (Duncan and Schulz, 2015; Lewis, 2014; Murray et al., 2015; Patterson et al., 2016). Although Giddens and Morton (2010) reported a drop in NCLEX pass rates with the first student cohort graduating from a concept-based curriculum, the authors noted a number of confounding variables (including a change in admission requirements, move from a 9-month to 12-month academic calendar, expansion of enrollment, and initiation of distance learning at an off-site campus) making it impossible to determine what role, if any, the initial drop of those passing was caused by the change to a concept-based curriculum. In a review of literature, Repsha et al. (2020) concluded that NCLEX pass rates, time to graduation, and graduation rates were not affected by the adoption of a concept-based curriculum. This is an important finding because of unfounded concerns shared by many faculty regarding curriculum change and the potential for poor program outcomes.

Standardized test measurements using Assessment Technologies Institute nursing education test scores and critical thinking assessment scores were used to evaluate the effect of conceptual learning in a concept-based curriculum compared with a traditional curriculum. The researchers found no statistically significant difference between the two groups but noted that the method of instruction may have moderated the effects of the concept-based curriculum (Fromer, 2017).

Time to graduation and graduation rates are other important curriculum outcomes. The concept-based curriculum did not change on-time graduation rates (Duncan and Schulz, 2015; Murray et al., 2015; Lewis, 2014), although two studies (Lewis, 2014; Murray et al., 2015) reported statistically significant improvements in program completion. Giddens and Morton (2010) reported a 97.5% graduation rate from the first three cohorts of graduates from a concept-based curriculum; however, there was no indication whether this was a change from the previous curriculum offered.

Program satisfaction commonly includes student and employer satisfaction. Several authors reported strong student satisfaction as measured in end-of-program surveys among those graduating from a concept-based curriculum, but these were not comparative measures (Gooder and Cantwell, 2017; McGrath, 2015; Patterson et al., 2016). Two studies reported no changes in student satisfaction as measured by an end of program survey (Lewis, 2014; Murray et al., 2015), whereas Duncan and Schulz (2015) reported lower mean satisfaction scores among the first graduating cohorts from a concept-based curriculum. Less information was reported on feedback from employers. Patterson and colleagues (2016) and Giddens and Morton (2010) reported positive feedback from the nursing community regarding student and graduate performance in clinical settings, while Lewis (2014) reported no changes in employer or alumni satisfaction.

Several other elements of curriculum evaluation associated with a concept-based curriculum are reported in the literature. These include:

- evaluating for "concept creep" (or, in other words, additional concepts being added to the curriculum) using a PDSA cycle (Laverentz and Kumm, 2017),
- improvement in students' critical thinking and/or clinical judgment (Duncan and Schulz, 2015; Harrison, 2018; Nielsen et al., 2021; Patterson et al., 2016; Repsha et al., 2020; Sportsman and Pleasant, 2017),
- higher order thinking (Getha-Eby et al., 2015),
- self-efficacy (Duncan and Schulz, 2015),
- students' perceived preparation to work in diverse clinical settings (Hensel, 2017),
- clinical competence among RN-BSN students in Taiwan (Lee-Hsieh et al., 2003), and
- student perceptions related to the quality of teaching/instruction among faculty in a concept-based curriculum (Gooder and Cantwell, 2017; McGrath, 2015).

Two other articles reported measures to ensure success for students enrolled in nursing programs with a concept-based curriculum. Barrett and Jacob (2021) reported on the success of a comprehensive support plan for accelerated students, while Pool et al. (2019) reported on ways to best support students with English as an additional language.

MISCONCEPTIONS AND CLARIFICATIONS

Misconception: There is an abundance of literature and evidence supporting the conceptual approach in the nursing education literature.

Clarification: Although the conceptual approach has been well represented in the education literature for decades, the same cannot be said for the nursing literature. Most articles published in the nursing education literature have emerged over the last decade. There is a need for ongoing robust educational research evaluating outcomes associated with conceptual learning.

ARTICLES DESCRIBING CONCEPT-BASED TEACHING AND LEARNING

A third general group of published articles in the nursing literature associated with the conceptual approach describes models or specific teaching strategies related to concept-based teaching or learning. Concept-based teaching refers to a process where faculty design learning activities that guide students through the study of one or more concepts, including unique aspects of nursing care related to that concept. It also involves a student-centered teaching approach with a variety of application-based learning activities.

As discussed in Chapter 6, conceptual teaching represents a departure from traditional, instructor-centered models of teaching. Thus the conceptual approach represents a transition for many nursing faculty members. Not surprisingly, faculty perceptions and experiences associated with the conceptual teaching approach have been a recent focus of research (Deane, 2017; Deane and Asselin, 2015; Pyatt, 2021; Sportsman and Pleasant, 2017; Wilhelm et al., 2020; Zhu et al., 2022). Common initial reactions experienced by faculty, as reported from these studies, include faculty feeling underprepared, loss of power, out of comfort zone, and a time-consuming process. However, common to the studies was a gradual process of acceptance and buy-in among faculty as they gained experience and saw benefits.

Concept-based teaching strategies have been designed for both clinical and classroom settings. In the clinical setting, the strategies are designed to help learners make connections between the concept, the nursing care, and patient outcomes as opposed to a focus the tasks of care associated with the clinical experience. Concept-based learning in clinical settings for nursing education was first reported by Heims and Boyd (1990), who reported improved learning outcomes when purposeful concept-based learning assignments were developed and applied in the clinical setting. Other articles describe the conceptual approach as a basis for linking clinical learning to the classroom (Nielsen et al., 2013; Nielsen, 2016).

The clinical judgment model is described as a foundation for concept-based teaching in the clinical setting (Lasater and Nielsen, 2009; Nielsen, 2009; Nielsen et al., 2021). Specifically, students focused on a specific concept for the clinical day; learning activities included study guides, patient rounds, and faculty evaluation and feedback. Authors reported that this approach increased direct contact time for students and faculty, with the opportunity for faculty to role-model communication, and allowed students to focus on one idea at a time. Authors also noted improvement in critical thinking as a result of concept-based learning in the clinical setting (Lasater and Nielsen, 2009). Hardin and Richardson (2012) describe a model of conceptual teaching in a concept-based curriculum. The core components of the model for effective conceptual teaching include addressing misconceptions, building enduring understandings, and developing metacognition. The authors also provide a description of five teaching methods proposed for effective conceptual teaching including misconception and preconception check, the discrepant event, concept maps, approximate analogies, and check your knowledge. Kantor (2010) describes the use of another model, the KBD approach (which stands for come to *know*, develop a way of *being*, and *develop* a plan of care) as a successful student-centered teaching and learning tool for linking clinical and classroom learning in a concept-based curriculum.

Several articles report on the use of the conceptual approach for specific topics or courses. Two articles presented a conceptual approach as a foundation for a capstone clinical course (Nielsen et al., 2021; Owens and Christian, 2021). Another article reported positive student feedback and a positive correlation of test scores after adopting a conceptual approach to a nursing pharmacology course (Lanz and Davis, 2017). The development of professional values was the focus of a study reported by Elliot, who found that students expressed an appreciation for a variety of professional values and a disillusionment with unprofessional values seen among some nurse (Elliott, 2017). The use of concepts in a professional development course was also reported by Nelson-Brantley and Laverentz (2014). Manning and colleagues reported on various ways infection is taught as a concept as a result of a review of the literature (Manning et al., 2020). Other topics featured in the literature include a concept-based learning activity to assess for amputation risk (Roach et al., 2021); teaching the concept of genetics (Elliott, 2019); immunity as a concept (Giddens, 2010); teaching informatics as a concept (Guerra, 2019); the course design and teaching of mental health concepts (Romanowski et al., 2021); transitional care (Mood et al., 2014); and social determinants of health (Decker et al., 2017; Porter et al., 2020). Two common themes noted among these included positive experiences among students and faculty, and also that faculty generally find the conceptual approach acceptable and or beneficial.

The concept map is perhaps the most recognized concept-based teaching strategy in nursing. Introduced in the education discipline in the 1960s by James Novak, concept maps organize information and show the relationship between ideas. This approach involves the integration of multiple ideas and concepts to extend the understanding. In nursing, concept maps show the relationship of concepts in the context of patient care, allowing the student to make important connections and learn interrelationships (see Fig. 7.1). A number of articles in the nursing literature feature concept mapping in the clinical and classroom setting (Alfayoumi, 2019; Aliyari et al., 2019; Chen, 2017; Harrison and Gibbons, 2013; Rahnama and Mardani-Hamooleh, 2017; Senita, 2008; Taylor and Littleton-Keamey, 2011); this strategy is credited with increasing student critical thinking and metacognition. A concept map development protocol was proposed as the result of a study conducted by Ab Latif and Mat Nor (2020).

Higgins and Reid (2016) reported the development of concept analysis diagrams for each concept in the concept-based curriculum, which then was used as a foundation for concept-based teaching in the classroom or clinical seminars. The diagrams show antecedents, attributes, consequences, and interrelated concepts and show how nursing care interfaces with the concept. Components of nursing care include assessment, analysis, intervention, and evaluation. Concept analysis diagrams differ from concept maps in that these are a visual representation of the concept as opposed to a learning activity where students draw a map showing interrelationships among concepts, usually in the context of a patient.

SUMMARY OF CURRENT LITERATURE AND GAPS

Based on the surge of published nursing literature during the last decade, an increased interest in the conceptual approach within nursing education is evident. The literature would also suggest that application of the conceptual approach is occurring primarily in undergraduate, prelicensure education and spreading to other countries. There are many variations in concept-based curricula; thus, these are not "cookie cutter" curricula; however, there are common attributes to all, including clearly identified concepts and exemplars. It is the organization of the concepts and exemplars within and across courses that vary.

One of the greatest barriers to curriculum reform is fear of failure and negative program outcomes. Faculty in some nursing schools may assume that if the NCLEX pass rates and other metrics (such as program completion and time to graduation) are "good," then there is little need for curriculum reform. The literature published to date suggests that changing to a concept-based curriculum does not negatively affect traditional program outcomes (NCLEX-RN pass rate, graduation rate, time-to-graduation, or student satisfaction). Findings also suggest that conceptual teaching practices lead to improved learning. These findings may be encouraging to faculty considering a change to the conceptual approach.

A variety of concept-based teaching strategies appear in the nursing literature—the most visible being concept maps. This area of literature should continue to evolve, so the evidence expands, and nurse educators have examples of best practices in concept-based teaching and learning. Traditional direct measures of program quality, teaching quality, and learning outcomes may not be sensitive to the true outcomes of the conceptual approach—in other words, the influence of the conceptual approach on clinical judgment, team-based care, and long-term patient outcomes. The next important step in scholarly work for the conceptual approach will be to tease out such differences if at all possible.

Developing Nursing Faculty Expertise in the Conceptual Approach

The conceptual approach is still in an early evolutionary stage in nursing. It takes time for a new method to be accepted and even longer for widespread proficiency among faculty to create optimal curricula with extensive and consistent incorporation of this approach into didactic and clinical courses. Most faculty are aware of the conceptual approach, and many nursing programs have recently adopted or are in the process of adopting this approach. Although an individual program has little effect on the profession as a whole, the collective effect of many nursing programs adopting the conceptual approach over time will lead to a tipping point by which we will begin to fully realize the benefit within the nursing profession.

Developing expertise in the conceptual approach requires a deep understanding of each of the interrelated elements—concepts, exemplars, concept-based curriculum, concept-based teaching, conceptual learning, and the evaluation of conceptual learning (including competency assessment). It is the integration of these components that leads to deeper conceptual understandings and mastery of the conceptual approach. These are not learned in a sequential or linear approach, nor can they be effectively learned in isolation. Gaining an understanding of the elements of the conceptual approach tends to occur together and over time. As nursing education evolves toward competency-based assessment, the intersection between competencies and the conceptual approach will become even more evident.

How do faculty develop skills and expertise in the conceptual approach? First, faculty members must be willing to shift their perspectives about teaching and the instructor role. The conceptual teacher might be best described as a *learning coach* who creates a learning environment where the focus is more on ideas than content, where the students are guided through a learning process in a way that stimulates synergistic thinking, and where the learners demonstrate critical reasoning and the ability to make generalizations. Many faculty have deeply rooted ways in which they view education and the learning process; the conceptual approach may challenge (or in conflict with) longstanding assumptions. Faculty must also be open to developing skills associated with competency assessment. Thus, being open-minded to learning, being open to the advice and suggestions of mentors, and being fully engaged and committed to ongoing professional development are needed to truly attain expertise. Let's face it; many faculty, particularly those who have been in nursing education for a number of years, pride themselves as expert teachers. Some may feel vulnerable with the adoption of a process they do not fully understand—thus, a natural reaction is to reject the idea. Feelings such as this are similar to those experienced by medical school faculty who have shifted to competency-based assessment (Sirianni et al., 2020). Thus, an environment must be fostered where these feelings and perspectives are acknowledged yet not allowed to derail efforts for curriculum and teaching reform.

MISCONCEPTIONS AND CLARIFICATIONS

Misconception: Most faculty successfully master the conceptual approach in a short period of time, especially if they attend a conference presentation or workshop.

Clarification: Achieving mastery in the conceptual approach takes time—even for experienced faculty. Gaining a general understanding of the conceptual approach must be followed by an ongoing commitment to implement and maintain the curriculum and dedicate themselves to applying conceptual teaching practices, seeking feedback, and actively reflecting on the process for self-improvement.

Professional development for faculty is the first step toward developing competence in the conceptual approach. The goals of professional development are to cultivate and increase an understanding of the conceptual approach and to extend expertise in conceptual teaching and evaluation of conceptual learning. Traditional approaches for faculty development include attending conferences or workshops on the conceptual approach. These approaches help to increase one's understanding and enthusiasm for change, but they are not often effective for successful and sustained change. Developing competence in the conceptual approach requires time, and thus it is not realistic to attend one presentation or workshop and "get it" (although it would certainly be convenient of this were the case). One learns to teach conceptually by doing it, learning from the experiences (both positive and negative), and then improving on those experiences. This is not a passive process! Proficiency is developed through the experience of applying principles associated with the conceptual approach and purposeful and deliberate reflection. This is usually most effective in conjunction with other faculty and mentors who are also committed (Sirianni et al., 2020). Erickson and Lanning (2014) specifically suggest establishing professional learning communities as an effective method to support faculty. Such communities can be formed among interested faculty within your school and colleagues from other schools or disciplines. Professional learning communities provide many opportunities for faculty to share ideas and experiences, to provide/receive feedback, peer evaluation, and coaching, or to discuss journal articles or books. Furthermore, such groups can provide suggestions or ideas for creative learning strategies, development of lesson plans, and evaluation process.

Attaining competence and expertise in the conceptual approach and skill in competency assessment is a developmental process whereby faculty progress from novice to expert over time. This process is truly a journey with an unspecified endpoint—meaning the developmental milestones are not specified at a fixed time or distance. Faculty on this journey will progress based on many variables, but perhaps the most important is being truly committed to the process. This requires openness to learning and dedicating the time and effort to a continuous process of learning, applying what has been learned, receiving feedback, and reflecting on the experience.

CONCEPTUAL APPROACH COMPETENCIES FOR NURSING FACULTY

It is one thing to be able to list the elements of the conceptual approach (concepts, exemplars, concept-based curriculum, concept-based teaching, conceptual learning, and evaluation of conceptual learning/competency assessment) and another to fully understand each element, how these elements are interrelated, and truly understand how the conceptual approach differs from traditional nursing education. Competencies are behaviors that provide a framework for faculty development and evaluation. Conceptual approach competencies for nursing faculty are presented in Box 9.1 and can provide guidance in professional development.

Beyond Nursing: The Conceptual Approach for Health Sciences Education

This book has been written primarily from the perspective of, and for the purposes of, adopting the conceptual approach in nursing education. However, the conceptual approach should be considered more broadly. Chapter 1 presented the background of the conceptual approach and traced its origins to the work of Helen Taba and the education discipline. Although unique concepts exist in each of the disciplines, concepts may also be applicable across multiple disciplines. This is particularly true among the health science professions.

BOX 9.1 ■ Nursing Faculty Competencies for the Conceptual Approach

Understanding, Support, and Rationale
Competency 1: Attains a Deep Understanding of the Conceptual Approach

- Articulates individual components of the conceptual approach.
- Describes how the conceptual approach differs from traditional nursing education.
- Explains the rationale, benefits, and challenges of the conceptual approach as a model for nursing education.
- Analyzes findings from research in nursing and other disciplines that support the conceptual approach.
- Engages in self-reflection related to teaching and demonstrates a commitment to ongoing professional development in the conceptual approach.

Concepts and Exemplars
Competency 2: Effectively Uses Concepts and Exemplars as Components of the Conceptual Approach

- Demonstrates a solid understanding of what concepts are, the common categories of concepts used in nursing education, and levels of concepts.
- Evaluates potential concepts using criteria for ideal concepts in nursing education.
- Differentiates concepts from exemplars and effectively links exemplars to the concept to deepen learners' conceptual understanding.
- Appreciates the value of using concepts as a way to frame nursing knowledge.

Concept-Based Curriculum
Competency 3: Designs, Implements, and Evaluates a Concept-Based Curriculum

- Applies change theories/strategies within the curriculum revision process.
- Engages and informs community partners and key stakeholders in the curriculum development process.
- Uses literature, research, and best educational practices to design and implement the concept-based curriculum.
- Clearly explains the curriculum, including how concepts and exemplars are organized and used within and across semesters and courses (didactic, laboratory, clinical).
- Develops measurable program outcomes and evaluates program effectiveness.

Concept-Based Teaching
Competency 4: Designs and Implements Lesson Plans That Incorporate Best Practices of Conceptual Teaching

- Develops lesson plans for classroom/didactic courses and clinical/laboratory courses.
- Concept units include a concept overview so that learners know what the concept is, understand the context of clinical practice, recognize the concept, and know what to do.
- Concepts are taught in a logical and consistent way, building on critical knowledge/facts and skills and incorporating guiding questions to facilitate conceptual understanding.
- Incorporates a variety of student-centered teaching strategies that align with learning outcomes.

BOX 9.1 ▪ Nursing Faculty Competencies for the Conceptual Approach
(Continued)

- Teaching strategies are intentionally designed to be interesting and challenging for student engagement and require learners to extend previously held knowledge to new situations, applications, and contexts.
- Exemplars and interrelated concepts are deliberately incorporated for a deeper understanding of the concept.

Conceptual Learning and Learning Assessment
Competency 5: Creates a Learning Environment That Optimizes Conceptual Learning and Achievement of Learning Outcomes/Competencies

- Demonstrates a solid understanding of the neuroscience of learning, including physiologic variables that affect learning.
- Creates a learning environment and fosters a learning process that is safe, stimulating, and rewarding.
- Challenges learners to make cognitive connections from previously held knowledge/skills to concepts, leading to synergistic thinking and the formation of generalizations.
- Uses a variety of strategies to assess student learning, competency attainment, and achievement of outcomes; learners demonstrate the ability to transfer information from one situation to another and can effectively solve problems.
- Demonstrates skill in performance assessments, coaching, and competency evaluation.

In 2003, the Institute of Medicine (IOM) published *Health Professions Education: A Bridge to Quality* (IOM, 2003) which called for health sciences education reform. It was recommended that five core areas be included in the education of all health professionals: patient-centered care, working in interdisciplinary teams, evidence-based practice, quality improvement, and information technology. These core areas are reflected as concepts in most concept-based curricula. In an update to this work, *The Future of Nursing: 2020–2030* reiterated the need to strengthen nursing education—this in part by incorporating competencies as a component of the curriculum and ensuring nurses are prepared to work collaboratively with other health and non-health professionals (National Academies of Sciences, Engineering, and Medicine, 2021). In 2011, the Interprofessional Education Collaborative (IPEC) created core competencies to guide curriculum development across the health professions, which were reaffirmed and refined in 2016. The IPEC competencies include teamwork and team-based practice, communication, values and ethics, and roles/responsibilities (IPEC, 2016).

To expand on this, multiple concepts such *Diversity* and *Inclusion*, *Professionalism*, *Health Policy*, and *Health Disparities* are found throughout the health sciences literature. All health professionals must also have an understanding of biobehavioral concepts such as *Gas Exchange*, *Mood*, *Mobility*, *Perfusion*, *Cognition*, and *Infection*, to name a few—the list could go on. What these concepts represent is the same but what truly differs is how each member of a health professional team interfaces with each other when the concept is represented in patient care. Put another way; there are variations in the roles and expectations of health care professionals—yet, all encounter the same set of concepts within their professional practice. This is not to say that the only difference between nurses and other health care professionals is the interventions, and in no way should this be interpreted as a diminishment of nursing as a unique discipline. Historically, nursing has had a significant role in health care delivery and is clearly established as a practice discipline.

MISCONCEPTIONS AND CLARIFICATIONS

Misconception: The concepts in a nursing concept curriculum are generally unique to the nursing discipline.

Clarification: Most concepts found in a nursing concept-based curriculum are actually applicable to all health sciences disciplines and could be considered as a foundation for interprofessional education. That said, nursing students enrolled in a nursing program offering a concept-based curriculum gain an understanding and application of the concept through the lens of professional nursing practice.

The case could be made for a conceptual approach to become the model for future health sciences education, especially considering the competency-based assessment movement in other health disciplines (American Association of Colleges of Nursing, 2021; Englander et al., 2013). It would be a natural way to support integrated interprofessional education experiences and concepts that also support competencies. Over the past decade there have been substantial attempts to incorporate interprofessional education in health sciences education; these have produced mixed results. The challenge of layering such experiences into existing and divergent educational structures of each discipline has made it difficult to achieve significant impact, as evidenced by the limited emergence of strong and efficient interprofessional practice models in health care. True interprofessional practice occurs when members of the health care team function in a way where all members are able to fully contribute to the care delivery using their unique knowledge and skills nested within the discipline that they represent, with the expectation of achieving optimal patient care outcomes. Although this occurs in some settings, it does not happen nearly enough. Most students today experience some degree of interprofessional education and may have an opportunity to be placed in a clinical setting where the optimal interprofessional practice is evident, but for the most part, these primarily remain as desired goals within the academic context. If the goal is truly to transform health care delivery through high-functioning teams engaged in interprofessional practice, health professions education must be aligned for that reality.

Summary

Nursing is leading the way in the adoption of the conceptual approach, and thus, nurse educators are well-positioned to lead education reform in health sciences education. There is a need for ongoing educational research associated with the conceptual approach in nursing education and other health sciences. Specifically, there is a need for the extension of best practices to support concept-based teaching and learning and more evidence regarding outcomes for learners and programs. With a growing emphasis on competency-based assessment, nursing has an opportunity to lead in this area by leveraging gains made in the conceptual approach through ongoing professional development; nurse educators should increase individual and collective expertise in the conceptual approach movement. Faculty have the ability to influence future generations of the nursing workforce equipped with higher-order thinking skills. With the evolution of concept-based interprofessional education, nursing faculty have the potential to extend their influence on students in other health care professionals and shape the future of interprofessional practice.

References

Ab Latif R, Mat Nor MZ. Using the ADDIE model to develop a Rusnani concept mapping guideline for nursing students. *Malays J Med Sci.* 2020;26(6):115–127. https://doi.org/10.21315/mjms2020.27.6.11.

Alfayoumi I. The impact of combining concept-based learning and concept-mapping pedagogies on nursing students' clinical reasoning abilities. *Nurse Educ Today.* 2019;72:40–46. https://doi.org/10.1016/j.nedt.2018.10.009.

Aliyari S, Pishgooie AM, Abdi A, et al. Comparing two teaching methods based on concept map and lecture on the level of learning in basic life support. *Nurse Educ Pract.* 2019;38:40–44. https://doi.org/10.1016/j.nepr.2019.05.008.

Allen P. Preparing nurses for tomorrow's healthcare system. *Am Nurse Today.* 2013;8(5):46–50.

American Association of Colleges of Nursing. *The Essentials: Core Competencies for Professional Nursing Education.* 2021. https://www.aacnnursing.org/Portals/42/AcademicNursing/pdf/Essentials-2021.pdf.

Barrett T, Jacob SR. A multifaceted comprehensive student success plan for accelerated BSN students in a concept-based curriculum. *Teach Learn Nurs.* 2021;16:169–174. https://doi.org/10.1016/j.teln.2020.11.003.

Brady D, Welborn-Brown P, Smith D, et al. Staying afloat: surviving curriculum change. *Nurse Educ.* 2008;33(5):198–201.

Brandon AF, All AC. Constructivism theory analysis and application to curricula. *Nurs Educ Perspect.* 2010;31(2):89–92.

Brussow JA, Roberts K, Scaruto M, et al. Concept-based curricula: a national study of critical concepts. *Nurse Educ.* 2019;44:15–19. https://doi.org/10.1097/NNE.0000000000000515.

Chen ZCY. A qualitative study on using concept maps in problem-based learning. *Nurse Educ Pract.* 2017;24:70–76. https://doi.org/10.1016/j.nepr.2017.04.008.

Christmasles CD, Crous L, Armstrong SJ. The development of concepts for a concept-based advanced practice nursing (child health nurse practitioner) curriculum for sub-saharan Africa. *Int J Caring Sci.* 2019;12(3):1410–1422.

Crookes PA, Lewis PA, Else FC, et al. Current issues with the identification of threshold concepts in nursing. *Nurse Educ Pract.* 2020;42:102682. https://doi.org/10.1016/j.nepr.2019.102682.

Deane WH. Transitioning to concept-based teaching: a qualitative descriptive study from the nurse educator's perspective. *Teach Learn Nurs.* 2017;12:237–241. https://doi.org/10.1016/j.teln.2017.06.006.

Deane WH, Asselin M. Transitioning to concept-based teaching: a discussion of strategies and the use of Bridges change model. *J Nurs Educ Pract*. 2015;5(10):52–58.

Decker KA, Hensel D, Kuhn TM, et al. Innovative implementation of social determinants of health in a new concept-based curriculum. *Nurse Educ*. 2017;42(3):115–116.

Duncan K, Schulz PS. Impact of change to a concept-based baccalaureate nursing curriculum on student and program outcomes. *J Nurs Educ*. 2015;54(3):S16–S20.

Elliott AM. Professional values competency evaluation for students enrolled in a concept-based curriculum. *J Nurs Educ*. 2017;56(1):12–21. https://doi.org/10.3928/01484834-20161219-04.

Elliott AM. An educational session to teach the concept of genetics. *J Nurs Educ*. 2019;58(2):122. https://doi.org/10.3928/01484834-20190122-13.

Englander R, Cameron T, Ballard AJ, et al. Toward a common taxonomy of competency domains for the health professions and competencies for physicians. *Acad Med*. 2013;88(8):1088–1094.

Erickson HL, Lanning LA. *Transitioning to Concept-Based Curriculum and Instruction*. Thousand Oaks, CA: Corwin Publishing; 2014.

Fromer RF. Theory-driven integrative process/outcome evaluation of a concept-based nursing curriculum. *Nurs Educ Perspect*. 2017;38(5):267–269.

Getha-Eby TJ, Beery T, O'Brien B, et al. Student learning outcomes in response to concept-based teaching. *J Nurs Educ*. 2015;54(4):193–200.

Giddens J, Brady D, Brown P, et al. A new curriculum for a new era of nursing education. *Nurs Educ Perspect*. 2008;29(4):200–204.

Giddens JF. Underestimated challenges adopting the conceptual approach. *J Nurs Educ*. 2016;55(4): 187–188.

Giddens JF. The immunity game: conceptual learning through learner engagement. *J Nurs Educ*. 2010;49(7):422–423.

Giddens JF, Brady DP. Rescuing nursing education from content saturation: the case for a concept-based curriculum. *J Nurs Educ*. 2007;46:65–69.

Giddens JF, Keller T, Liesveld J. Answering the call for a bachelors-prepared nursing workforce: an innovative model for academic progression. *J Prof Nurs*. 2015;31(6):445–451. https://doi.org/10.1016/j.profnurs.2015.05.002.

Giddens JF, Morton N. Report card: an evaluation of a concept-based curriculum. *Nurs Educ Perspect*. 2010;31(6):372–377.

Giddens JF, Wright M, Gray I. Selecting concepts for a concept-based curriculum: application of a benchmark approach. *J Nurs Educ*. 2012;51(9):511–519.

Gooder V, Cantwell S. Student experiences with a newly developed concept-based curriculum. *Teach Learn Nurs*. 2017;12(2):142–147.

Goodman T. Nursing education moves to a concept-based curriculum. *AORN J*. 2014;99(6):C7–C8.

Guerra D. Teaching clinical informatics in a concept-based flipped classroom. *Nurse Educ*. 2019;44 (3):129–131. https://doi.org/10.1097/NNE.0000000000000586.

Hardin PK, Richardson SJ. Teaching the concept curricula: theory and method. *J Nurs Educ*. 2012;51 (3):155–159.

Harrison CV. Predicting success for associate degree nursing students in a concept-based curriculum. *Teach Learn Nurs*. 2018;13:135–140. Doi: 101016/j.teln.2018.01.005.

Harrison S, Gibbons C. Nursing student perceptions of concept maps: from theory to practice. *Nurs Educ Perspect*. 2013;34(6):395–399.

Heims ML, Boyd ST. Concept-based learning activities in clinical nursing education. *Nurs Educ Perspect*. 1990;29(6):249–254.

Hendricks S, Wangerin V. Concept-based curriculum: changing attitudes and overcoming barriers. *Nurse Educ*. 2017;42(3):138–142.

Hensel D. Using Q methodology to assess learning outcomes following the implementation of a concept-based curriculum. *Nurse Educ*. 2017;42(5):250–254.

Herrington A, Schneidereith T. Scaffolding and sequencing core concepts to develop a simulation-integrated nursing curriculum. *Nurse Educ*. 2017;42(4):204–207. https://doi.org/10.1097/NNE.0000000000000358.

Higgins B, Reid H. Enhancing "conceptual teaching/learning" in a concept-based curriculum. *Teach Learn Nurs*. 2016;12:95–102.

Hollinshead J, Stirling L. A conceptual curriculum framework designed to ensure quality student health visitor training in practice. *Community Pract.* 2014;87(7):22–25.

Institute of Medicine. *Health Professions Education: A Bridge to Quality.* Washington DC: National Academy Press; 2003.

Interprofessional Education Collaborative. *Core Competencies for Interprofessional Practice: 2016 Update.* Washington DC: Interprofessional Education Collaborative; 2016.

Kantor SA. Pedagogical change in nursing education: one instructor's experience. *J Nurs Educ.* 2010; 49(7):414–417.

Lanz A, Davis RG. Pharmacology goes concept-based: course design, implementation, and evaluation. *Nurs Educ Perspect.* 2017;38(5):279–280.

Lasater K, Nielsen A. The influence of concept-based learning activities on students' clinical judgment development. *J Nurs Educ.* 2009;48(8):441–446.

Laverentz DM, Kumm S. Concept evaluation using the PDSA cycle for continuous quality improvement. *Nurs Educ Perspect.* 2017;38(5):288–290.

Lee-Hsieh J, Kao C, Kuo C, et al. Clinical nursing competence of RN-to-BSN students in a nursing concept-based curriculum in Taiwan. *J Nurs Educ.* 2003;42(12):536–545.

Lewis LS. Outcomes of a concept-based curriculum. *Teach Learn Nurs.* 2014;9(2):75–79.

Manning ML, Pogorzelska-Maziarz M, Ward J. Infection concept integration and teaching strategies in US baccalaureate nursing programs in an era of concept-based curriculum. *Nurse Educ.* 2020;45 (5):E45–E49. https://doi.org/10.1097/NNE.0000000000000767.

McGrath B. The development of a concept-based learning approach as part of an integrative nursing curriculum. *Whitireia Nurs Health J.* 2015;22:11–17.

Mood LC, Neunzert C, Tadesse R. Centering the concept of transitional care: a teaching-learning innovation. *J Nurs Educ.* 2014;53(5):287–290.

Murray S, Laurent K, Gontarz J. Evaluation of a concept-based curriculum: a tool and process. *Teach Learn Nurs.* 2015;10:169–175.

National Academies of Sciences, Engineering, and Medicine. *The Future of Nursing 2020–2030: Charting a Path to Achieve Health Equity.* Washington, DC: The National Academies Press; 2021. https://doi.org/10.17226/25982.

Nelson-Brantley HV, Laverentz DM. Leaderless organization: active learning strategy in a concept-based curriculum. *J Nurs Educ.* 2014;53(8):484.

Nielsen AE. Concept-based learning activities using the clinical judgment model as a foundation for clinical learning. *J Nurs Educ.* 2009;48(6):350–354.

Nielsen AE. Concept-based learning in clinical experiences: bringing theory to clinical education for deep learning. *J Nurs Educ.* 2016;55(7):365–371.

Nielsen AE, Lanciotti K, Garner A, et al. Concept-based learning for capstone clinical experiences in hospital and community settings. *Nurse Educ.* 2021;46(6):381–385. https://doi.org/10.1097/NNE.0000000000000964.

Nielsen AE, Noone J, Voss H, et al. Preparing nursing students for the future: an innovative approach to clinical education. *Nurs Educ Pract.* 2013;13:301–309.

Owens RA, Christian SJ. A hybrid concept-based clinical practicum course: an innovative approach to baccalaureate nursing education in a rural area. *Nurs Educ Perspect.* 2021;42(6):E105–E106. https://doi.org/10.1097/01.NEP.000000000000823.

Patterson LD, Crager JM, Farmer A, et al. A strategy to ensure faculty engagement when assessing a concept-based curriculum. *J Nurs Educ.* 2016;55(8):467–470.

Pool L, Day L, Ridley S. Mountain climbing: the journey for students with English as an additional language in a concept-based nursing curriculum. *Whitireia J Nurs Health Soc Serv.* 2019;26:28–36.

Popoola M. Popoola holistic praxis model—a framework for curriculum development. *West Afr J Nurs.* 2012;23(2):43–56.

Porter K, Jackson G, Clark R, et al. Applying social determinants of health to nursing education using a concept-based approach. *J Nurs Educ.* 2020;59(5):293–296. https://doi.org/10.3928/01484834-20200422-12.

Pyatt A. Lessons learned: implementation of a concept-based curriculum in the development of a new prelicensure nursing program. *Nurs Educ Perspect.* 2021;42(6):E103–E104.

Rahnama F, Mardani-Hamooleh M. Iranian nursing students' perceptions regarding use of concept mapping: a concept analysis. *Res Dev Med Educ*. 2017;6(1):45–50. https://doi.org/10.15171/rdme.2017.008.

Repsha CL, Quinn BL, Peters AB. Implementing a concept-based nursing curriculum: a review of the literature. *Teach Learn Nurs*. 2020;15:66–71. Doi: 101016/j.teln.2019.09.006.

Roach A, Lloyd-Pena M, Wallace S. An innovative concept-based learning activity to identify and educate veterans at risk for amputation. *Nurs Educ Perspect*. 2021;42(6):E131–E132. https://doi.org/10.1097/01.NEP.000000000000779.

Romanowski A, Allen P, Martin A. Educational revolution: integrating concept-based curriculum and active learning for mental health nursing students. *J Am Psychiatr Nurses Assoc*. 2021;27(1):83–87. https://doi.org/10.1177/1078390319890031.

Senita J. The use of concept maps to evaluate critical thinking in the clinical setting. *Teach Learn Nurs*. 2008;3(1):6–10.

Sirianni G, Takahashi SG, Myers J. Taking stock of what is known about faculty development in competency-based medical education: A scoping review paper. *Med Teach*. 2020;42(8):909–915. https://doi.org/10.1080/0142159X.2020.1763285.

Sportsman S, Pleasant T. Concept-based curricula: state of the innovation. *Teach Learn Nurs*. 2017;12:195–200. https://doi.org/10.1016/j.teln.2017.03.001.

Taylor LA, Littleton-Keamey M. Concept mapping: a distinctive educational approach to foster critical thinking. *Nurse Educ*. 2011;36(2):84–88.

Trossman S. A change in the air? Nurses discuss value of a concept-based approach to education. *Am Nurse*. 2015;47(4):1–10. http://www.theamericannurse.org/2015/08/31/a-change-in-the-air/.

Wilhelm S, Rodehorst-Weber K, Longoria A. Transitioning from a traditional to a concept-based curriculum: faculty's experience. *Nurs Educ Perspect*. 2020;41(6):355–357. https://doi.org/10.1097/01.NEP.0000000000000562.

Zhu Y, Pei X, Chen X. Faculty's experience in developing and implementing concept-based teaching of baccalaureate nursing education in the Chinese context: a descriptive qualitative research study. *Nurse Educ Today*. 2022;108:1–6. https://doi.org/10.1016/j.nedt.2021.105126.

Note: Page numbers followed by *f* indicate figures, *t* indicate tables, and *b* indicate boxes.